Disease Detectives:

Case of the Pink Snake

By David M. Owens

Introduction

Welcome to public health as it's been practiced for decades. Regardless of whether you are new to public health or a life learner who's curious about what we do, I'm certain that you'll learn some important lessons from this book. Experienced investigators will enjoy a nostalgic, or commiserative, journey through these pages. Public health professionals without a patient care background will improve their understanding of field investigations.

The story follows Scott, a veteran disease investigator, and Sara, the rookie, through a short sexually transmitted disease investigation. Sarah and Scott encounter interesting patients, social situation, and behaviors throughout and apply innovative and time tested techniques to aid them in their goal. Due to the content and language this book is not appropriate for young readers.

I wrote this book to emphasize the importance of what's called "traditional partner services". That is, public health workers who go into the community to educate people and gather information so that they can stop disease outbreaks. There are those in public health who question the effectiveness of this approach. But having performed traditional partner services for many years I can attest to its continued reliance and importance.

The stories related in this novel are based on encounters that my coworkers and I have had over the years. Obviously events, names, and locations have been changed to protect the confidentiality of the patients. Any similarities to known events or names are purely coincidental. Also, the investigative practices have been altered for the sake of the narrative. This book is not designed to be a how to book on conducting field investigations as much as an introduction to partner services for those who are interested in the social aspect of public health investigations.

I have a disclaimer. The views and opinions expressed in this novel are my own. They do not represent those of the State of Kansas or any of it's agencies, the US Armed Forces, the Centers for Disease Control, or any local governments or health departments.

Prologue

Scott closes the manila folder filled with forms and notes, lab results, and post-its that occupies the center quarter of his small desk. He opens one of the four file cabinets that sets near his modest desk glancing over the numerous similar files until he locates the "M" section. He divides two folders and positions the most recent folder between them. "Another case closed" he tells himself. Taking only a short moment to reflect on the lives touched, the situations presented, the challenges faced during the last investigation, Scott takes in a deep breath and closes the file drawer. He notices that the number of files has grown considerably over the last couple of years. Each represents an infected person and the people they were with. Each file containing the unique, but predictably similar stories that lead to them acquiring the disease; and in some cases spreading it to their loved ones.

The medium framed man in his late forties with graying hair sits in a small office, in an old building that houses the community's only public health clinic. Scott has an unremarkable appearance with medium length hair and features. His dress is static business casual attire, dull solid colors, and off brand articles. He wears only a modest brown and silver watch and no jewelry. A pair of silver rimmed glasses acts as the dominant feature on his face.

Scott is one of the few disease investigators at the public health department. His official title is "Disease Intervention Specialist", a cold but efficient name for a person who spends his day keeping people from getting and spreading disease, mostly sexually transmitted. Scott began disease intervention almost fourteen years ago when he left his job at a for -profit laboratory.

The office where the detective works is adorned with a diverse collection of memorabilia collected over his lifetime. A hat from his high school, pictures of college friends; bags and name tags from the various conferences he attended over the years hang in corners collecting dust. They are seldom viewed or reflected upon, but their presence allows him to keep track of what this middle aged public servant has done. A person does not easily become something, they are made into that by their choices and experiences. Scott's experiences and choices brought him to this place from an odd path.

Scott had been a good student in high school. He was dedicated to his studies and balanced his academic obligations with a spirited social life. He was rarely without a girlfriend and many male friends. His wit, easy going personality, and accepting friendly nature attracted people to him. He found people fascinating. The way they interact, the way they make decisions, and how they deal with the inevitable consequences of those decisions was of great interest to him. He studied his friends, teachers, and the other adults around and learned a lot from observing them. Early on, Scott became aware of the value of quietly listening to people to acquire sensitive information about them and others. Sure, questions are great, but often someone would tell him all he needed to know if he just listened to them long enough.

Scott knew he liked interacting with people, but like many children and young adults, he struggled with finding his niche. Realizing that the medical field offered both financial security and a multitude of employment options, Scott entered college with the intention to become a clinical therapist. Conducting therapy would allow Scott to use the skills he acquired through years of observation. It would also allow him to assist people who, in many cases, desperately needed the attention. It wouldn't hurt that he would make a pretty good living too. That thought, through daydreaming, always brought a slight smile to his face and was often followed with dreams of the proper dispensing of his fictional, though anticipated, wealth.

At the state university Scott majored in Chemistry and had every intention of applying to the clinical psychology program after completion. He interned at a small lab during his last year and was offered a position after graduation. It was a good job and thought it steered him away from his goal of counseling, was still helping people. He gladly accepted.

Scott's parents were supportive of their middle child's endeavor. He came from a middle class family where both his mother and father worked in the public sector. They both graduated from the local state university and actually met while attending there. Scott's mother was employed as a manager at the city's Department of Revenue. She worked there until her retirement a few years ago. His father worked for the Water Department. The two provided a safe comfortable home for their three children. But Scott's father often worked late and when he did come home was tired and moody. He was an unhappy man who drank consistently, but seldom to excess, Scott remembers the routine consisting of the man walking in the door, briefly greeting the family members who had already eaten, and going to the shower. He would emerge from the shower and get a beer, a plate of dinner, and recline on the large chair in the common room. There he would watch television, seldom acknowledging the family and never initiating the interaction, until bed time.

Scott didn't want to live like that. He wanted to have fun, enjoy his work, and come home to a loving family. He wanted that white picket fence that is the American dream. But the more he watched, he realized that the reality is more complicated.

His own attempt was perhaps a greater failure than his parent's willingness to reside in mediocrity. Scott divorced twelve years ago after just a few short, but painful years of marital purgatory. His marriage did provide him with two daughters, Ellisa and Monica. His ex-wife, Scarlet, kept the girls after the divorce. Scott sees them every other weekend or so, when they don't have something better to do. Teenagers can been hard to keep up with and slightly self absorbed. Still, Scott cares from them very much, and keeps a picture of them in his office.

Of the many problems with the marriage, Scott fell into the same rut as his father, even after promising himself that he would never allow himself to have the joy of life sucked from him by a job or interpersonal conflict. Scott came home from the work late. He would shower and go into the kitchen, get a beer from the refrigerator. His wife and the children may or may not have been there, but there wasn't anything prepared for him to eat. He would usually warm some leftovers from the previous day or get a bowl of cereal. Scott's physique had deteriorated into a moderately overweight flabby mess. His muscular slender build covered by the consequence of a sedentary life. He didn't feel like he had any energy, and looking back on it, he now knows he was depressed.

His wife filed. She was tired of him not being there emotionally. Scott had to concede that she was right to leave and since the separation and subsequent divorce, life has improved for everyone involved. She remarried a couple of years later and the new husband is a good man. He's bonded with the girls much better than Scott did. It seems his white picket dream was attainable after all.

After a few years of his single life spiraling into obscurity Scott decided to make a change. He started by exercising and changing his diet. He now feels better than he had in years. He took up yoga and Bujinkan for relaxation and exercise. Through his study of meditation and martial arts he realized that he had separated from his path and needed to again find his way in life. He felt his career was stagnant and lacked purpose. Boredom was the order of every day and though he made a decent living, Scott wanted more than money. He got into the medical field to make a difference in people's lives, to better society. At the laboratory the routine was killing him. He began searching the classifieds for a new career.

A college friend of his, Ann, had been working at the local health department as a nurse. During a dinner with her and her husband she suggested that he apply for a disease investigator position there at the clinic. Scott was initially unsure about making the change. The job seemed odd. Why would the government pay someone to do what doctor's offices should be doing? Besides, people with sexually transmitted diseases could easily inform their own partners to get treated. And the pay was, well, not an incentive. The whole idea sounded ridiculous but something about the career intrigued him. The thought of getting back into a field where he would work intimately with people addressing sensitive situations for the betterment of both the individuals and the community as a whole was appealing. So Scott applied.

During his interview the director, Shawn Epps, told Scott that he would work with patients with many different problems all going on at the same time. Those problems overlapped, and in some cases synergized causing dysfunction on a scale not often seen by lay people or even doctors. The patients Scott would work with would have problems including illegal drug use, prostitution, sexual abuse, psychological disorders, poverty, poor education and many others. The task seemed overwhelming. Scott asked during the interview why the doctors couldn't contact the patient's partners, or at least have the patients contact their own partners to get them treated. Shawn laughed at this question. "Doctors do health care. We do public health." The answer seemed vague to Scott at the time, but now, after working in the trenches for years it is as obvious to him as it was to Shawn all those years ago. We do public health.

Chapter 1

In a large apartment complex near downtown a woman is heard screaming obscenities at her lover. "God dam Mutha Fuck'r, you dirty…" A tall lean man wearing a dirty t-shirt and badly stained jeans responds to the assault. "Look Bitch, don't you be try'n to act like I won't woop your ass. Keep talk'n shit." Red's tone and demeanor encourage her to reduce her hostility, but she continues to express her displeasure with the current situation. "You should have told me. What the Fuck?!" The calm that follows is short lived. A crash of a thrown porcelain lamp, a couple of loud heavy foot steps at a run, the subtle hollow thud of a naked fist striking flesh is followed by more screaming.

The woman in the apartment across the hall huddles with her two children in the love seat, fearful of the altercation that transpires so close to her home. Each violent outburst resonates within her as she recalls her own tragedy. Upon hearing the final screams her resolve bolsters and she frees her cell phone from its charging area. "911 Emergency…"

The building returns to its usual auditory state offering a symphony of footsteps, televisions, light conversations, with a spattering of children playing in the court just beyond the main entrance. The police cruisers appear quickly and converge on the building with beautifully coordinated precision. The officers patiently approach the apartment and find the beaten woman sobbing on a chair in the front room. Broken furniture and decorations lay scattered in the once peaceful room that is now racked by violence. Of the three police responders, Officer Mac enters the apartment first. The woman stands to greet the police and conveys her version of the dynamic incident which led to the destruction of her home. "He gone now." She asserts with conviction. "I kicked his ass out, he aint going to hit on me no mo'." "Where is he now?" inquired Mac, as he ran though the possible hideouts in his mind. "Don't know, don't care…long as he stay the hell away from me." The victim regains some of her tenacity. "You haven't been smoking rocks tonight have you Mrs. Johnson?" Mac's ample experience with this couple gives him an insight into the situation that a casual viewer would likely miss. "No sir, I've been clean for four months." The woman lies without hesitation maintaining eye contact throughout. "What about Eddie? Was he using before all of this?" Mac realizes the answer prior to asking the question, but uses this to gauge her honesty.

"Yes, he's been in the streets every night for weeks. He come home late, high, and I duno how he pay for it."

"Are you going to press charges this time Mrs. Johnson? You know he's going to keep hitting you if you let him back in here." The middle aged woman becomes quiet and appears introspective. Inside she wrestles with knowing that the officer's words are true. But Eddie provides the money for her to survive and losing that stability is more than she can manage now. "Na, he aint com'n back."

The officers excuse themselves and stroll somberly back to their cruisers. Mac suspects that Eddie is at Grungy's house getting high and waiting for the police to leave so he can return to the apartment. Mac calls in and completes his paperwork on the incident in time to receive another call from a distressed citizen, another domestic, another familiar name

***

The county public health clinic is located downtown near a small shopping center that contains a Radio Shack, dry cleaners, a used furniture store, and a Mexican food restaurant named La Cosina. The latter is a favorite for the employees of the clinic for lunch and occasionally post work dinner and drinks. The Health Department is in an older building, having first been a department store, then a Department of Motor Vehicle annex, and later still a Social Security office. After the site no longer met the needs of those organizations, it was given to the county health department to relocate them closer to the community that they serve. It was debatable whether or not this new site is an improvement from the previous. But the location does have the advantage of being centrally located and accessible by public transportation. Both of those reasons were sufficient to justify the move.

The building itself has a light brown brick exterior with large windows. It has two above ground levels and a basement. The structure has a large independent parking lot with wheelchair ramps leading to each entrance/exit. Blue and yellow signs identify the building as the local health department.

The first floor is where the patients are seen by the clinic staff. The front entrances lead immediately to the reception desk and waiting area. There are several exam rooms along the exterior walls behind the reception desk. The main floor also contains a small laboratory near the center of the level. The laboratory has a refrigerator, a few microscopes, a counter with sinks and many cabinets which contain a variety of medical supplies. A large room just behind the reception desk houses the patient medical records. This room is filled with filing cabinets which are themselves filled with manila patient charts. There's been considerable discussion concerning modernizing to an electronic medical record system, but that has not been implemented as of yet. The rest of the first floor is taken up by support staff offices to include the administrative assistant, supervisor, the social worker, the nurses' office, and the disease investigator offices.

On the second floor are administrative offices, the employee lounge, and a large conference room. The director's office is in one of the corners, child care licensing and restaurant inspection staff share another corner office. The county epidemiologist (epi) has a space right next to the lounge, which is in a corner near the bathrooms. The conference room is located in the center of the floor and contains a large wooden table in the center of the great room. It is largely devoid of furnishings other than the chairs and some audio visual equipment.

The information technology office, storage, maintenance, and bio-terrorism are located in the basement. Some call it the dungeon because the lighting is substandard in the halls and the walls are a stone gray. But the offices are well lit and, other than the lack of a view, comfortable and roomy.

***

"Scott, this is Sara." The introduction is presented by the clinic director. Scott looks up from his computer monitor and greets the couple. "Good morning Ann, nice to meet you Sara. Welcome aboard." Scott vaguely recognizes the young woman from her interview a few weeks ago. So many have come and gone it's become difficult to remember all of the faces let alone the names. Ann is a slender woman in her mid forties. She always carries herself with confidence and has a distinct air of professionalism. "Scott, I need to meet with you when you get a moment, please." Even her instructions were toned and phrased with class and professionalism to extend a persona of competence and genuine concern for her clinic. "I'll be there in five." Scott responds. Sara provides a forced smile, "Nice to meet you Scott." "Likewise." Scott responds with an easy grin that seems genuine, but contains a hint of nostalgic irony.

Meeting new people reminds him of his own first walk around the clinic. Scott reminisces briefly, and then rubs his face in surprised recognition of the obvious. "Not many of those first day faces are still here." He tells himself. Peggy, the enduring public health nurse, who's been a staple of the clinic since as far back as anyone can remember; and Ann who was a public health nurse herself before moving up to administration. Scott smiles at the memories, and then closes down his computer. He retrieves a pad of paper and a pen from the top of his desk and leaves his office to meet with Ann.

Ann's office is a large room, well lit and decorated modestly. File cabinets, book shelves, and office equipment line the walls, while above them are scattered picture frames mostly presenting achievements and recognitions the director has gathered over the years. A large bordered picture frame acts as the centerpiece of the collections. Large print at the top reads "University of Kansas." Smaller picture frames on her book case and desk contain pictures of family members, friends from school, and work. One picture depicts Ann receiving an award from the governor. Scott smiles when he sees it. "Isn't this the guy we voted against?" he said playfully. "He still helps pay the bills, Scott." She rebuts. "How's William, did he get his knee fixed yet?" Scott inquires about Ann's husband. "No...he's hard headed and thinks it'll fix itself."

Scott takes a seat in the old leather chair across from the director. "What can I do for you, boss?" "As you know, Sara is the new DIS, and I want you to mentor her. I believe that you have a lot to teach, and your experience would be a real asset in her training." Ann locks her fingers together in front of her face as she makes this directive. "My pleasure." Scott responds but his mind scrolls through all of the cases he needs to work and realizes that training a new person will certainly slow his progress. Scott excuses himself and leaves the office to locate the rookie.

Chapter 2

"This is some bull shit!" Red lifts the corner of the blinds to peer out of the window. "Quit fuck'n with my window bitch. No tell'n who's look'n in" Grimy exclaims before he inhales from a small glass pipe. White smoke escapes his nostrils after a few seconds of inhaling the crack. Grimy, a skinny short man in his twenties could easily pass for a man in his late thirties. His home is a haven for characters of ill repute who seek an escape from the difficulties of lower class urban life through consumption of illegal narcotics. Grimy provides them with that escape, but at the high price of their ability to function effectively in society.

"Shit man, I can't go back right now. You know I've got warrants." Red replies in an agitated tone with matching demeanor. "Can't believe that bitch called Five-O on me. She's got to be tripp'n." Grimy shoots Red a disgusted look, "Mutha fuck'r you need to get your shit straight. Keep your mind in the game." A woman enters the room wearing short shorts and a bra. She has a tattoo of paw prints ascending her left thigh. She looks like she's in her early twenties, but she has the aura of an older woman. "Yo bitch." Grimy motions to the young woman. "Come over here and suck my dick." The young woman approaches him and gets on her knees in front of the dealer. Grimy smiles and lays back on the couch. "See partn'a, this is the shit. This is what bitches is good for."

***

Scott approaches Sara's office. He peers though the door and sees her unpacking a small cardboard box. "I see you're settling in nicely." The tone is upbeat but received with a melancholy response. "It's fine. I have everything I need, thank you." Her response is cold, but cordial. Sara removes some items from the box and places them around the bare office. A few small pictures, a couple of statuettes and some office supplies are removed and placed on the desk which serves as a staging area for the various office accommodations. Among the items is a diploma framed "Colorado University...Masters of Public Health..."

"Congrats on your graduation Sara, is this your first real gig?" Scott chuckles at the jest, but Sara coldly glares at him.

"I was in a dual MD/MPH program, but didn't complete med school." Sympathetic, Scott replies "Sorry, are you going back?" "I started an application to University of Kansas, with any luck I'll get accepted for next term." Scott, still sympathetic "Best of luck, I hope you make a fine physician. In the meantime, this job isn't so bad. You'll get to see some things that most doctors don't." Showing a fake smile Ann replies "I look forward to it." No longer smiling Scott rebuts, "Well, we'll be working together. Come see me when you're done unpacking and we'll start your training."

***

"What do you think of the new girl?" Fully realizing that Sara is in her early twenties, the director phrases the question to reflect her view of Sara's experience rather than her age. "I think she's overqualified for this." Scott responds without hesitating. "She has a Masters in Public Health from Colorado, applied to their med school, and she appears to be on her way up the ladder."

"Well…an entry level disease investigator position wasn't her dream job after school, but with the economy being such as it is…we are fortunate to get her." Scott laughs "We'll be fortunate to keep her." Ann concedes the point, with a nod and a subdued hand gesture. "She's a very bright young woman, I expect that she'll do well." Scott sits on the end of the desk "If she wants to…I agree." Ann's desk phone rings signaling the end of the meeting. "Sorry Scott, I need to get this." Scott stands and excuses himself. "This is Ann, …yes…"

***

"How may we help you?" The emergency room triage nurse asks Mrs. Johnson. "My stomach hurts real bad, I need to see a doctor." Mrs. Johnson is distressed and nearly doubles over. "Your name, miss?" the heavy set nurse in light blue scrubs inquires without lifting her eyes. "Chris Johnson" the anticipatory patient replies. Making eye contact with the new patient and using her vast experience she briefly assesses her, "Please complete this and have a seat in the lobby, we'll get to you shortly." The nurse hands the new patient a clip board with several blank forms attached. Wincing, Mrs. Johnson accepts the forms and slowly walks to the padded seats facing the front desk. She eases into a chair and begins completing the forms. Minutes seem like hours as the agony persists. She places the clipboard next to her and bends over to gain just a little relief.

"Mrs. Johnson?" the nurse calls, "you may come back now." The nurse's words are welcome and the young woman stands and follows her back to a room prepared for her in the emergency department. The pair pass through the automated security doors and a large open work station buzzing with activity from medical staff and biomedical equipment. Chris is brought to the room where she hopes to receive relief. The small room feels cold. An exam table is situated in the center against the wall. Numerous medical machines and a few cabinets are against the walls. "Please slip this on," the nurse hands Chris a hospital gown and in her best presentation of a well-used medical cliché "The doctor will be with you shortly." Chris removes her clothing and slips on the fragile garment. She sits at the edge of the exam table with her legs crossed and her hands folded in her lap. Again, time slows as she awaits the arrival of the physician.

***

Light enters the room through the small opening in the aluminum foil which covers the windows. It touches Red's face and spurs him awake. He sits up from the couch where he's been sleeping and surveys the large living room. The house is full of people still, but few are stirring. Feeling his bladder full, Red rises and staggers to the bathroom. Along the way he steps over a few of Grimy's customers who are propped against the hallway walls and laying on the floor. The stink of unwashed bodies, uncleaned facilities, smoke, and stale air cause Red to frown. Chris kept our place clean by comparison. He missed home briefly but the filthy bathroom was a welcome site. Red unzips his pants and as he began to relieve himself an intense pain accompanies the stream of dark urine. "Aaaaaahhhh!" Red struggles through the pain to finish the act. He puts his penis back in his stained underwear and secures his jeans. Breathing hard and invigorated by the experience he views his hazy reflection in the dirty mirror. Red turns the valve on the sink and cold water spews forth allowing him to rinse his face. "I got to get this shit looked at." Referencing the time on his fake Rolex, ten forty-two, Red concludes that the clinic should see patients at this time. He exits the bathroom, bounds down the stairs and leaves Grimy's home. He finds his twenty-three year old Lincoln parked where he left it outside. The engine requires some prodding and encouragement, but eventually turns over allowing him to drive to the county health department.

***

"No, the black boots go with that much better." Sandy argues with James at the front desk of the clinic. James views the picture on the computer screen. "If you want to look like a hooker." Sandy's lips pucker in a hurt look and she cuts her eyes at her co worker. "Whatever, my friends agree with me." James laughs, "so we're not friends now?"

The clinic door opens and Red walks through. He cautiously approaches the counter. Sandy greets the patient with a perky tone and a smile, "Good morning Mr. Johnson." She recognizes Red from his multiple previous visits to the clinic. "I need to see the nurse" Red announces to the receptionist. "You don't have an appointment sir, I'll have to make you one…hmmm" Sandy views the computer screen which now displays the clinic schedule. "Can you come in on Thursday at three thirty?"

"Naw, I got to see her now!" Red exclaims in an agitated tone. Scott overhears the conversation at the reception desk and comes out to talk with the patient. "Hi Red, can you come back to my office?" Red and Scott walk a short distance and enter Scott's office. "What's going on?"

"That bitch burnt me again" Red asserts. Scott replies, "We got you treated a couple months ago when you had gonorrhea. How many people have you been having sex with?" Offended, Red replies "Just my wife, man. The meds must not have worked."

Scott maintains a calm demeanor even though he's frustrated by the situation. "Remember when I said that we have to get all of your partners treated or you'll get it again? Now you're telling me that she isn't sleeping with anyone else, so if that's the case than you are. Look, when I contact your partners I don't tell them anything about you, no names, no dates, no locations. But I need know who you've had sex with so we can get them taken care of. That way you don't keep getting this." Red's expression mutes and his shoulders fall slightly. "Alright, there's this other one, but I don't know her real name." Scott nods careful not to act either surprised or judgmental. "That's fine Red. Let's start with what you do know. What name does she go by?" "Peaches."

"How old is Peaches?"

"She about twenty two."

"What does Peaches look like."

"She about five five, thick, got hair that come down to her back."

Scott nods as he writes down all of the information in carefully practiced format. "What's Peaches phone number?"

Red shrugs "I ain't got it."

"So how can I get in touch with her?" Scott inquires. Red gestures indicating that he doesn't know. Scott thinks for a moment and lets the silence dominate the room. After several moments Red reveals that he meets Peaches at Grimy's house a few times a week. Scott follows up with several more probing personal questions which make the patient very uncomfortable. In time Red admits that he gives Peaches crack to have sex with him.

Scott knows Grimy's name very well, but has not had the pleasure of a meeting. He thinks that Grimy may have come into the health department several months back while Scott was in the field. But all attempts to reach him have ended in failure and none of the many people who've become infected and named him as a partner would talk about how to find him. Red's information was no different.

"Well Red, I'll ask the nurses to take care of you today. I want to get you tested so we know exactly what we are dealing with."

"Man I got to get that shit stuck in my dick again?" Red grimaces remembering the urethral swab from previous exams.

"Yes, but with all the discharge it shouldn't hurt. Also, I want to get some blood from you to test for syphilis." Scott reassures Red.

"Syph-a-what?"

"Syphilis, Red. It's a very dangerous disease. It's curable, but if you have it and it goes untreated can destroy your heart, lungs, brain...basically it can maim you and can eventually kills you."

"But it's curable...that's good."

"Also Red, we are going to do a test for HIV."

"I ain't got no HIV!"

"With HIV you may not have any symptoms for years so the only way you'll know if you're infected is if you get tested. HIV isn't the death sentence it was back in the 80's because of the new medications that are available, but if someone has it and doesn't get meds they can still get very sick and die."

"Man I don't want no HIV test."

"Red, the thing about HIV is that you either have it or you don't. If you have it you want to know so that you can get on meds, if you don't have it you want to know that you don't have it. This test is going to give you the information you need."

"Alright man, when do I get my shot? I got shit I need to do."

Scott smiles, "Let's go see the nurse."

***

A woman enters the emergency room wearing medium blue scrubs and with a white identification card affixed to her top "What brings you to the hospital Mrs. Johnson?" Dr. Anderson briefly greets the patient. "My stomach hurts" responds the reluctant patient.

"How long has this been going on?" The physician sits on a backless stool on wheels and rolls closer to the patient. "A few days…" Chris underestimates to the doctor. "OK, well let's take a look. Can you lay back on the table?" The debilitated patient lays back and the doctor begins her examination of the young woman.

***

"Ok Red, the nurses did a Gram Stain and you tested positive for gonorrhea. They are going to send your tests to the state lab for additional testing, but we are going to get you treated before you go."

"Oh man! Not again. Airight, let's do this." Red girds up his loins for his non invasive injection and small pills that will control the infection. "Let's talk about your other partners first, Red" Scott suggests.

"Man I already told you." Red asserts with conviction.

"Yes, but I don't believe that those are the only ones. I need to know about all of them so we can stop the spread of this disease. It may seem like gonorrhea isn't a big deal, Red, because we can give you a shot and some pills and make it go away. But the fact is that it can be very dangerous for women who are infected. It can make it hard for them to have children later and cause long term pain. The infection can even get into the blood and infect other organs in the body causing some serious health problems."

"Aint nobody else." Red claims again. Scott nods realizing that the infected man is self absorbed and not concerned with the welfare of the women that may be affected by this disease. "Ok, Red. If you do think of anyone else just give me a call." Scott hands Red a business card from his pocket and asks if the patient has any questions about the infection. He educates him about ways to protect himself and the dangers of sexually transmitted diseases like Gonorrhea, Chlamydia, Syphilis, and Human Immunodeficiency Virus. Scott then excuses himself and exits the exam room.

After a few moments a middle aged woman wearing scrubs adorned with cartoon characters enters Red's exam room. "Hi Red. I hear you're not feeling so well." The tone is pleasant with just a hint of facetiousness. "Are you ready for your shot?" Red grimaces and gets to his feet. He undoes his jeans and exposes a butt cheek. "Ahhhhhhh!"

Scott looks up from his desk upon hearing the patient call out. "It's a little shot mixed with lidocaine, doesn't even hurt." Scott says to himself. He shakes his head and resumes typing on his computer. Scott uses a program specifically created for public health infectious disease monitoring to manage the many cases he's working. He identifies three more cases of gonorrhea that have been assigned to him. Opening the files he views the first and locates the phone number. Scott lifts the receiver from its cradle and dials the doctor's office that reported the first case. "Thank you for calling

Clear Lake Clinic, Debbie speaking, how may I help you?"

"Hi Debbie, this is Scott at the health department. How are you?"

"I'm fine, it's been busy here lately. Who are you calling about?"

"You guys have another gonorrhea patient that I need to get treatment on and talk with, her name is Jenny Switzer."

Recognizing the name and knowing that Scott would call about this patient, nurse Debbie replies "Oh ya… poor thing. She was treated at time of service. Her address is…" The nurse gives Scott the information he needs to find the young woman and hopefully prevent her from getting infected again. The process is repeated for the next two patients. "Thanks Debbie, talk with you again soon." The conversation ends and Scott organizes his newly acquired information and prepares to locate the recently diagnosed young people.

Scott prints some letters for each of the patients. "Oh wow, the day's gone by fast." Scott tells himself as he glances at the clock. It's fifteen till five. He turns off his computer and the small light over his desk. Grabbing his backpack and his jacket, Scott leaves his office and makes his way to Sara's office. "Hey Sara" Scott enters her space as she is preparing her belongings for the post day exodus. "Good, you've got your things ready. We're headed out." Sara, clearly taken off-guard by the late intrusion and confused by the statement fails to respond. "We're going to find some disease" Scott informs her.

Ann passes them in the hall, "Leaving early?" she inquires with a slight smile. "I need to do some field visits on the way home." Scott holds up the envelopes to show his boss. "Be careful and see you tomorrow." Ann replies in her usual polite tone. "Thanks, see you tomorrow." Sara offers a halfhearted wave to her boss and follows the mentor through the hallway. The duo exit the building and walk to his car, Scott carrying his bag over one shoulder. He locates his late model four door Ford economy car and unlocks the doors with the remote. Scott tosses his bag in the backseat and takes his seat in the trusty vehicle. He notes that usually his stuff rides shotgun so he has easier access. It's rare to have anyone accompany him in the field. With map in hand, Scott starts the car and drives towards the first house on the list. He hopes the patients will be home, but in case they aren't he'll leave the letters for them to contact him tomorrow.

Navigating his well used vehicle through neighborhoods, business districts and more neighborhoods, Scott arrives at a small blue house. He parks the car a house down from the one identified as belonging to the sought after patient to avoid suspicion. The home has a small wooden porch with a few children's riding toys in the front. There are bars on the windows and a red Chevy Impala parked in the small drive directly to the left of the house. The car has dark windows and large wheels that create an unnatural ground clearance.

Scott gathers his notes and affixes them to a clip board that he stored in the pocket behind the passenger seat. He places the envelope on the clip board and checks his rear view mirror for traffic before opening the door and leaving the car. Sara gets out of the car and follows Scott. The spikes of her high heels sink into the yard as she walks awkwardly. Long experience has shown Scott that arriving at the door with a clip board is received much better than with just the envelope. He's found that an envelope by itself is associated with legal actions such as warrants, legal summons, eviction notices, and bills. People will often look outside and see the envelope in his hands and not come to the door. Whereas, the clip board makes him appear more like a delivery man, repair person, or sales representative. Curiosity is a better motivator to get people to answer the door than fear.

Observing the surroundings and patiently approaching the home, Scott notices that the blinds are all down and closed in the windows. The front door is closed. He can hear a television on inside the house. As he approaches the porch, Scott notices a chain that's used to tie up a dog and some food. He doesn't see a dog, but makes a mental note to watch for one. Scott approaches the front door and knocks loudly so that the summons can be heard over the television. A small dog is heard barking inside the home for a while then becomes quiet suddenly. Scott knocks again. No barking is heard this time. Scott realizes that the occupants have silenced the animal in an attempt to avoid contact with him. He places the envelope in the screen door, sticking out a ways so that it is visible from the street. The two investigators exchange a look and they return to the car.

Scott hands the clipboard to his passenger, starts the vehicle, and pulls away. He drives down the street watching the house in his rear view mirror. He takes a right at the end of the block, takes another right at the end of the next block, then another, then another. The investigators arrive back at the house to find that the letter he left in the door has been removed. Scott points out the sign to his protégé and places the car in park in the same location as before. "Sometimes it's the simple tricks" He smiles, collects the clipboard from the passenger, and the two approach the house again. Loudly knocking on the door again, Scott patiently waits for a few moments. Soon a young woman opens the door and meets Scott's gaze.

"Good afternoon. Is Ms. Rose Drake here please?"

"Yes" the young woman says in a quiet voice. "Who are you?"

"My name is Scott, and I'm with the county health department. Can you tell me what your date of birth is so that I can verify your identity?"

"May sixteen…" she replies.
"Thank you. I need to talk with you about the positive lab test for gonorrhea you received from your doctor's office last week. What do you know about gonorrhea?"

"My doctor said it's a sexually transmitted disease and it can go away with the shot and pills I got."

"That's true" Scott replies. "But it's still very dangerous. "If you get the infection multiple times or stay infected for too long then it can cause some serious problems for you." Scott goes on to educate her about the complications of the infection to encourage her to both get partners treated and to avoid reinfection. The young woman acts receptive to the information Scott is providing for her and seems genuinely concerned about her health. But she's conflicted.

"Who's the last person you had sex with, Rose?" Scott inquires. The pause tells Scott that she may be weighing the benefits verses the perceived social problems involved with disclosing this sensitive information. "When I contact them I don't tell them anything about you. They'll never hear from me that you gave me their information. And I really do need to talk with them so that they can get treated and not give you this infection again."

The logic is inescapable and the young woman is swayed by the argument. "I don't know his real name, but he goes by Red." Scott realizes the annoyed feeling welling up in his gut, but makes a conscious effort to maintain a flat affect. "Where is Red living?" The young woman provides Scott with directions to Red's apartment building where she meets him occasionally when his wife is away.

"Who else have you had sex with in the last couple of months?" Rose is taken off guard by the question, but responds by providing two other names of guys in the area. "Pritchard Wallace, and Dustin Evens." They are both friends of Red and Scott is familiar with Pritchard. "Dustin just got out." Rose offers. "He's staying at a half way house by the high school."

"Thank you very much for all of your cooperation with this Rose. I know this is a lot of personal information and it's hard to talk about." Scott offers his sympathies. "It's OK, I just want to make sure I'm safe." Rose responds.

"So who else?" Scott inquires. Rose is taken aback for a moment. "I did it with Grimy once a couple weeks ago at a party." Rose, clearly embarrassed, admits to the encounter. Her body language and facial expression tell Scott that she doesn't think that was a good idea.

"OK, I want you to know that I'm not here to judge you. It's my job to try to stop the spread of disease by getting people treated. You're doing a good thing by letting me talk with these guys. "So who else?" Rose shoots Scott an offended look and asserts "That's it. There isn't anyone else." Scott educates the young woman about risk reduction and gets ready to leave.
"Well thank you very much, Rose. Here's my card. If you think of anyone else or have any questions please call me."

Sara quietly takes in the whole experience and actively processes the many facets. She smiles and nods to the patient and turns back towards the car ahead of Scott. Scott opens the door and stares down the street for a moment. "Grimy…" He says to himself. "I've got to find this guy." He'll have another chance at it tomorrow.

***

"Well, it looks like you have pelvic inflammatory disease, Mrs. Johnson." The doctor presents the information in a very matter of fact tone and as easily as if it had been spoken by an actress who's script was well rehearsed. "What's that mean?"

The patient acts surprised, but doesn't quite pull off the role with conviction.

"Pelvic inflammatory disease, or what we call PID for short, is a bacterial infection in the uterus and/or fallopian tubes." The doctor removes a flip chart from a nearby table with pictures of the internal female anatomy to help describe the condition. "When the bacteria get past the cervix and enter the uterus it can cause the type of pain you are describing. The infection can even spread to the fallopian tubes." The doctor uses a pen to point to the locations she's talking about. "When this happens the body responds by building scar tissue which can cause you to experience long term pain. Sometimes that scar tissue can block the tubes and prevent the eggs from reaching the uterus. If that happens than it'll be very difficult, if not impossible, for you to conceive a child."

"I've already got two kids, don't need no mo. But can you get rid of it?" The patient responds. Dr. Anderson reassures her that the proper testing will be performed and that they will identify the cause of the pelvic inflammatory disease. "It's possible that the infection is caused by gonorrhea and/or chlamydia. Is your sex partner having any symptoms?"

"I don't think so." The patient lies to the physician.

"Well, it's best that he gets checked out too. A lot of times guys don't have symptoms, but it's still important that he gets taken care of. You don't want to get this again do you?"

Unfortunately this isn't Mrs. Johnson's first run-in with sexually transmitted disease. She's been infected before and blames Red for causing her so much pain and embarrassment. She's angry, but with everything going on knows she can't leave him.

"We should get your test results back shortly but I'm going to go ahead and treat you now. We'll also give you something for the pain. You should feel better in a few days." Dr. Anderson gets up from the stool and exits the room. On her way out, the patient calls to her. "Thank you Doctor." Smiling and truing her head to face her, Dr. Anderson graciously responds. "You're welcome."

***

Scott drives while using a well practiced combination of maps, street recognition, and global positioning system (GPS) from his smart phone to reach the desired location. They arrive at the address. The patient is supposed to live in a building at a large apartment complex on the west side of town. It's a nice enough place, clean and well maintained. Usually the visitor parking is just outside the main office, but after driving around the complex Scott isn't able to find the office. He does eventually find the visitor parking and deposits his car in an empty spot. Scott again retrieves his clipboard and his referral letter from Sara and they both get out of the car. The wind picks up a little bringing the temperature down to a brisk level. The cold air causes Scott's joints to stiffen a little. "I'll need a Motrin when I get home" he says to himself. He looks through the back window of the car and sees a light jacket dangling from the seat and resting on the floorboard. Scott opens the back door and retrieves the garment. Sara, already prepared for the possible inclement weather is wearing a red wool pea coat with a belt that trails freely behind her. Scott sets the clipboard down on the roof of the car and puts on the jean jacket, buttoning up most of the buttons. "Much better" he comments. With the impact of the cold weather addressed Scott and Sara walk towards the sprawling apartment complex. He locates the address easily enough, 1915, not far from where he parked. One side of the complex is labeled 101 through 114, 201 through 214, 301 through 314, 401 through 414 and 501 through 514. The apartment he is looking for is 418 so he walks to the other side of the building. As usual, no elevator is equipped for this building so they climb the many stairs to the fourth floor. They walk down the exterior open hall and locate apartment 418. The blinds are closed and no sounds are heard from within. A mat lays at the entrance just outside the door and a pair of old shoes loiter to the side. A couple of cigarette butts were inconsiderately discarded near the entrance. He looks for security cameras outside the apartment that would belong to the tenant. Wireless web cams, or for the more cost conscience paranoid person, web cams with wires are often used to monitor the entrance of a residence. Scott doesn't see any. What he does see indicates that someone does live at the apartment, though the lack of activity in conjunction with the time of day indicates that the occupants may not be home. He knocks at the door with four loud bangs and listens closely. Scott positions himself so that he can see all of the blinds at the front of the apartment simultaneously. Sometimes people will open the blinds to see who is knocking at the door before deciding to open it. If he can make eye contact at that time it makes it more likely that they'll answer. But no such luck. He knocks again and waits. Sometimes waiting for a few moments can result in making contact. But no one comes to the door and Scott slips the referral into the crack between the door and the frame. Scott turns and looks out over the wooden guard rail onto the rest of the apartment complex. He notices a building in the center of the large court yard that appears to be a multipurpose structure. A pool adjoins the building along with a brown shed. The two descend the steps and approach the building. There is a sign for a maintenance section and a main office. Walking around the building to find the door marked "office" Scott opens the door and is greeted by a young woman behind a large wooden desk. "Welcome to Greenwood Properties, how may I help you?" the young lady asks with a smile. She's wearing a red blouse with shoulder length hair. No wedding ring. Scott notices the latter out of reflex not interest. "Hi, my name is Scott and I'm looking for Angie Small in apartment 418. Is she still there?"

"I'm sorry sir, I'm not allowed to give out information about our residents." The young woman loses her smile, but remains friendly. "That's completely understandable" Scott assures her. "But it's really important that I talk with her. You don't have to tell me where she is, I just need to know if she still lives here." They young woman swayed by Scott's persistence and professionalism assumes that the business is official. She types briefly on her computer then reports to Scott that the person does live there, but she's a couple months behind and is pending an eviction. "Thank you very much." Scott excuses himself and he and Sara leave the apartment management office. This news disturbs Scott, because the patient will duck the management of the building. She may not be there at all during the day and may in fact have already moved. Scott looks at the apartment from the courtyard and sees that the envelope is still in the door. They walk back to his car.

Scott removes his smart phone from his pocket after reaching the car and Google searches the patient. Numerous possible entries are listed in the browser including a Facebook link. Scott smiles "Everyone has Facebook these days." And young people are great at updating it constantly. Often times with their location or with where they plan to go and when. The investigator accesses the Facebook page and begins scrolling through her posts. Most of it is the usual self absorbed young person testimonials, but there was a change in her status from "Single" to "in a relationship". She also indicated that she is talking about moving in with the new found love interest. Again, Scott smiles. He locates the page for the boyfriend and writes down his name. Scott locates the young man's date of birth, what school he's going to, and where he works. "It's amazing how much information young people put on these sites." Scott sends her a message on Facebook stating that he has very important health information he needs to discuss with her. He leaves his phone number on the message and closes his smart phone. Scott opens the door to the car and climbs in again. The clipboard is passed to Sara and he looks up the address of the next patient. It's not too far from here and this should be it for the day.

Sara realizes that she needs to let her dog out and that she's already working an hour past her time to get off. She anxiously monitors her watch hoping that Scott will quickly conclude the day's lessons. Scott parks in front of a two story white bungalow with a five foot high chain link fence that surrounds the property. The covered porch is cluttered with outdoor furniture, trash bags full of unknown items, and faded broken miscellaneous children's toys. He gets out of the car and greets his student. "This is the last one" he assures her. She doesn't respond, but her body language and facial expression tell him she's relieved. The couple walk up the few steps leading from the curb past the sidewalk and to the cement walkway interrupted by the chain link fence. Scott walks up to the fence and looks around. He then rattles the fence and waits for a long moment. After being sure that a dog is not somewhere in the yard Scott unlatches the gate and enters the yard with Sara right behind him. She turns to close the gate. "Leave it open" Scott directs the young investigator. "We want to keep our exit clear." Sara does as he asks and they approach the house. Scott again remains observant for any changes in the house due to their presence. He knocks on the door and then waits patiently, listening and watching the home for signs of movement. After what seems like a long moment for Sara, footsteps are heard approaching the door. A high school aged boy with sweats and shower shoes answers the door and looks out from inside the house through the screen at the two. "Hi, my name is Scott and this is Sara, we are looking for James Jefferson." The boy responds "That's me, who are you?"

"We are with the health department. We are here because one of your sex partners tested positive with gonorrhea and we would like for you to come down to the clinic to get tested and treated."

"I aint got noth'n" replied the teen.

"I'm not saying that you do, just that you've been exposed. It's possible to have gonorrhea and not have symptoms so I really suggest that you get treated at a minimum." Scott goes on to educate the boy about the infection. "What time would you like to come in tomorrow?" Scott sometimes sounds more like a sales person than a public health worker. "I got to be at school by eight thirty, don't get off till three thirty." He attempts to create a schedule conflict. "Perfect" Scott energetically replies "We can see you at four."

The patient reluctantly accepts the treatment appointment. Scott writes the time on the back on a business card and hands that to the young man. "Here's the time, on the other side of the card is the clinic address and my name and phone number. If you have any questions or need anything don't hesitate to call me. I'll be in the office at eight."

He accepts the card "OK, thanks." He closes the door.

Scott looks at Sara, she looks drained, fatigued. Being in the field energizes him because it allows him to do the job the best way he knows how. "Do you have any questions?" Scott asks.

"Why do we come out here? Wouldn't it be easier to just call?"

Scott smiles "We have to meet the patients where they are. It's much easier for them to ignore a phone call than someone who is standing at their doorstep ringing the bell. And we've got to contact people in order to get a handle on the spread of disease. Knocking on doors is a big part of how we do that. Sure, it's time consuming and expensive. But there's no substitute for shoe leather epidemiology." Sara gave Scott a confused look. "Shoe leather epidemiology?" she repeated. Scott anticipated the reaction. "Phones, internet sites, mail all have their place in this job. But many of the people we need to find don't want to be found. Some avoid us because they think we are bill collectors, law enforcement, sales people. Some people know that they are infected or at risk but they are just scared and don't know how to get the help they need. So we come to their homes, work, schools, hang outs, or anywhere else we can find them so that we can get them the information they need and encourage them to seek care. That's one of the things that separates us from the clinics, hospitals, and doctors' offices. We don't just let people fall through the cracks. Out here" Scott points around the neighborhood "is where our work is. The theologian John Wesley once said, "The world is my parish". Well, I'll borrow that idea and say that the world is my clinic." Scott spreads his arms wide and tilts his head back while gesturing towards the outside.

Scott can tell that Sara isn't sold on the idea and he gets the impression that the last point was a little over the top. It may have been how she rolled her eyes after the world…clinic statement. Still, Scott made his point and she had to concede that going to the field was, at least occasionally, useful.

The two return to their cars and bid the other good night. Tomorrow would provide another chance to learn and save lives.

***

Scott sits in his car for a moment. He calls the clinic to leave a voice message for the receptionist to set up an appointment for James to get treated. He completes some light paperwork and places his forms and clip board into a soft shell brief case and places the brief case on the floor of the passenger seat. He takes a sip of cold coffee from the travel mug in the cup holder on the console. It's just something wet to drink. Then he starts the car and points it towards home.

Chapter 3

About fifteen minutes later Scott arrives at a moderate sized apartment complex where he lives. He moved here after the divorce. It was supposed to be a temporary move, but he's liked the low maintenance apartment living and found the area convenient and much quieter than most. Shopping centers and a good bar and grill, the Angry Gator, are within walking distance. The complex has an indoor pool, hot tub, and sauna that are open year round. Scott parks his car in the carport labeled with his number. He walks up a flight of steps and down a hall to get to his home. "What a day" he comments to himself. Scott's apartment is well decorated with a variety of items that represent his varied interests. There are a couple of full bookshelves with novels, religious texts, reference books, and a few text books that he chose not to sell after completing the college class. Pictures of his children are sporadically placed around the living and dining areas, which are adjoined by a mock wall with an unnecessary, but decorative high arch.

Scott sets his keys, pocket knife, bill fold, clinic identification badge, and pens into a tray next to the door on his way in. He hangs his jacket on the hook by the door and takes off his shoes. He enters the small kitchen area and washes his hands. Opening the refrigerator he removes some left over spaghetti that Patty made for the two of them a couple nights ago. The spaghetti is put into the microwave and Scott retrieves a beer from the refrigerator and opens it. The sound of air escaping the bottle as it is opened is a very welcome sound and the liquid being poured into his mouth is like a little piece of heaven. Scott turns on the one of the burners on the stove top and fills a sauce pan with water and frozen vegetables. After a couple minutes the spaghetti is warmed up, the vegetables are boiled, and the beer is half gone. Collecting his meal onto a plate, Scott finds his way to his chair where he sits down and begins to enjoy his meal, vaguely bothered by some discomfort under his rib cage. He adjusts and it mostly goes away. He turns on the TV and watches the tail end of the six o'clock news.

During the program Scott's phone rings. "Hi baby, what's up?" Scott answers. Patty responds with a loving tone that Scott very much appreciates. "Not much, was just thinking about you."

"You're sweet, how was your day." He continues on with the small talk.

"I'll have to tell you about it in person. What are you doing tonight?" Patty inquires with a hint of self invitation.

Scott doesn't object "No plans, want to come over?"

"Give me about thirty minutes sweetie." Patty states. "See you soon, good bye."

Scott puts his plate down on top of the coffee table and gets out of his comfortable chair. He loves spending time with Patty, but her coming over means that he needs to tidy up a bit to avoid embarrassment. Scott spends the next twenty minutes gathering dirty dishes and putting them into the dish washer, picking up his dirty cloths and putting them into the hamper. He does an abridged bathroom clean up, and straightens up his room.

Lighting some incense is the final step to mask any estranged odors that may come from his apartment. The smoke permeates the whole domicile filling it with sweet smell of the black mountain forest. He wonders if the black mountain forest really smells like this, but the thought quickly escapes when he hears his doorbell.

Scott opens the door with a glass of wine in his off hand. "Hi sexy, you're early." He hands her the glass which she gratefully accepts. "Did I give you enough time to clean up or should I come back in a few minutes?" She jests with Scott.

"My place is always clean." Scott pretends. They both laugh and Scott pulls her close and kisses her. Holding hands they walk over to Scott's couch. "So what's going on?" Scott prepares himself for the detailed explanation of her latest drama at work. Patty, who is a nurse at the local hospital intensive care unit, loves her work. They met at her hospital when Scott came to interview a man who appeared to be dying from AIDS. She was the nurse on the floor at the time and they both realized the chemistry early on.

"There was another motorcycle accident." Patty said with a wince.

"Was he wearing a helmet?" Scott asked, but he already suspected that he wasn't.

Patty shook her head slowly. "I don't know why these guys don't wear helmets."

Scott thought back to his work saying, "Probably the same reason my patients don't wear condoms."

Patty continued her description of the patient. "I worked intensive care today and they brought the guy over from the emergency room. Scott…" she paused for a moment "the road rash stripped away most of the skin on his face and down the whole right side of his body. The surgeons will begin the skin grafts tomorrow if they can stabilize him."

"That is horrible. Is he going to make it?"

"We don't know yet. Maybe. But even if he does the head trauma and other injuries are so bad that he won't make a full recovery. He'll be lucky to be functional."

Scott's heard enough of these stories to know that "functional" means going to the bathroom on his own, dressing and feeding himself. This guy will probably never work again. Someone will have to take care of him for the rest of his life. However long or short that may be.

"And he has a family." Patty continues. "His wife and three month old child came up to the ICU shortly after he got there. She stayed for a while, but had to leave to take the child home. No one else came to see him so I don't think he has other family in the area." Patty kicks off her shoes and puts her feet on couch. She places her head against Scott's chest with his arm around her. He kisses her forehead and rubs her shoulder.

"I'm sorry. Legislators should have passed those helmet laws. Motorcyclists think they are free and invincible, but when they fall off of those bikes and high speeds…it just doesn't end well." Patty, done talking about the incident sips her wine, a delicious moscato.

"Do you want me to put in a movie?" Scott offers his guest.

"You didn't tell me about your day. How's the new girl?"

"Smart, but doesn't want to be there. If she gets past that she could be a good investigator." Scott isn't much of one to talk about work. Even if something is really bothering him. And while he understands his girlfriend's desire to discuss her job, his preference is to leave his at work.

Conceding that she won't get much else out of Scott she changes the subject back to the evening's entertainment. "OK, what movies do you have? Nothing with ninjas."

"Well that eliminates about half my movies. What about killer robots?"

"No."

"Aliens?"

"No."

"Something with love and lots of talking?" Scott laughs and she smiles. "Sure, what is it?"

"Aliens verses Ninjas…"

"Yuck, No! you're making that up. There is no such movie."

But Scott shows Patty the video case and she views it in disbelief. The terrible quality of his movie collection is almost enough to make her reconsider her association. She smiles at him but shakes her head declining the suggestion.

The couple agrees to watch an old James Bond movie, Goldfinger. It's a classic from a cinematic golden age. Scott retrieves a blanket from the hall closet and joins Patty on the couch again. They cuddle and enjoy the movie till it ends and the hour grows very late.

After the movie Scott turns to Patty who is almost asleep. "Are you staying?"

She looks at Scott's face "Of course." He stands and takes her hand to help her up. Scott turns off the TV and the lights in the living room and checks the lock on the door. They walk to Scott's room and turn off the lights.

***

Scott's alarm goes off way too early. It's still dark outside and it's cold. "I don't want to get up." Scott cuddles his girlfriend. "Me either, let's just call in and lay in bed all day." Patty says with the covers over her face.

"OK." Scott agrees, knowing he's got to go into work though.

"I can't." Patty, realizing the demands of responsible adulthood pulls the covers off of her face. She reluctantly climbs out of bed. She retrieves her bag from the floor near the bed and enters the small three quarters bathroom just outside of the bedroom.

Scott sits up and surveys the room. Still groggy from staying up too late he swings his legs over the bed and places his feet on the cold floor. The shock of frigid wood is sent through his body jolting him to greater consciousness. He feels around the side of the bed with is foot in search of his house shoes and locates one. The other must have been pushed beneath the bed. Scott gets down on all fours to look under the bed for the missing slipper instantly locating and retrieving it. The brief morning exercise lifts even more fog from his mind and Scott shuffles to the kitchen. "Hay baby, do you want some coffee, cereal?" Scott calls to Patty through the thin apartment walls. "Just some cereal, and fruit if you have any." Patty calls back from within the bathroom. The shower is running creating a splendid white noise throughout the small apartment. Scott pours a bowl of low sugar health food cereal in a couple of bowls and places a banana next to each. He pours a couple of glasses of carrot and tomato juice and sets those on the small circular dining room table. Patty is a health food enthusiast who's been working with Scott to improve his diet. The rabbit food isn't bad once he got used to it. But he'd love a stack of pancakes with bacon and cheesy scrambled eggs. "Mmmmm" Scott dreams about the breakfast he could be enjoying. Then he looks down at his bowl of oats with nuts and dried berries next to his fruit and his glass of vegetable juice and sighs. It's for the best, he tells himself.

Patty emerges from the bathroom dressed and ready for work. "Where did you keep your clothes?" Scott inquires, not remembering a suit case when she arrived. "Ladies secret." She says as she approaches the table where the health food feast has been prepared. The couple sits and talks while they eat. Occasionally holding hands or touching each other with their feet.

Shortly after eating Patty gets up from the table "I have to go." Her voice is sad but playful. "I know. Me too. I should get ready for work soon." Scott leaves the table and walks Patty to the door. They kiss and he gives her a final hug before she departs. The apartment becomes still with her gone. Scott leaves the dishes on the table; he'll get to them later. He showers and dresses in about fifteen minutes and leaves the apartment shortly after her.

***

Scott arrives at the health department just as the clinic is opening. "Good morning." He greats the reception staff cheerfully. "How are things going?"

Sandy responds first "I'm fine, glad it's Friday." James seconds the sentiment with a nod then takes a sip of his coffee.

"What are your weekend plans?" Scott asks as he stops at the reception desk. The desk is actually a collection of desks, tables, and carts. There is an impressive collection of computer terminals, fax machines, copiers, phones, printers, and other office gadgets to facilitate the managing of patient flow and record keeping. The receptionists are often among the first employees at the clinic. They'll make sure the lights are on, the doors are unlocked, and that the janitors haven't messed up anything over the night. It's a very demanding job with a long learning curve. The workers who sit behind this desk are invaluable members of the clinic team. And James make great coffee.

One of the roles that James took on is that of clinic coffee brewer. James used to be in the Army and credits his military experience for his ability to make the strongest pot of coffee the civilian community has ever experienced. Nothing less than a full cup of grounds goes into his special brew infusing the liquid with caffeinated goodness. James takes another sip of the coffee. "Sweet nectar of the gods," he expresses his approval for his creation.

***

James' Army career began the same way most recruits did. During high school he wasn't sure what path to take. He'd taken a few semesters of high school recruit officers training school and liked it well enough. Shortly before graduation the recruiters came calling.

First it was Chief Petty Officer Carter, a burly man with a hard face and a chest full of ribbons. The ribbons were impressive to behold, but the meaning was lost on a boy with limited experience. Chief Carter told James all about the adventures that he'd have as a seaman in the Navy. The fact that the Navy thought it was ok to call enlisted men (and women) seamen was, in James' underdeveloped opinion, an egregious oversight. The following ranks, petty officer third class, second class, and first class were no more appealing. "What is a petty officer" James wondered. "Is it like an officer, but not a very good one?" And the uniforms were, well, not as nice as some of the others. And what's the deal with that white hat that looks like an upside down dog bowl? After careful consideration, James decided that spending months at a time viewing nothing but water and gray paint wasn't for him.

Likewise James was approached by Sargent Benjamin of the United States Marine Corps. James liked the Marines dress uniform a lot. It was certainly the best looking one of all of the branches. Sargent Benjamin spoke highly of the Marine Corps and about courage and commitment and something else that James couldn't remember. But he was taken aback when he realized that the Marine Corps wouldn't tell him what he'd be doing if he enlisted. "So I won't know what my job is until after I sign up?" James was suspicious. He liked the idea of the Marine Corps, but remembered watching movies like Full Metal Jacket and Platoon where Marines, many of whom didn't sign up for it, became infantry men and endured miserable conditions before being extinguished in combat and dying horribly. "The uniforms aren't that nice" James thought to himself.

Sargent Downing from the Army spoke with the cadets at the high school ROTC and gave them information about the Army. The Army is a large organization with many different careers available. James liked the idea of flying Predator drones. He'd seen them in action on the news during the Middle East wars and since he was already familiar with flying radio controlled aircraft it seemed a natural fit. So James agreed to take the Armed Services Vocational Aptitude Battery (ASVAB) and enter the Army as a private first class. He was a good student in high school so it's no surprise that James did well on the test. He went to the Military Entrance Processing Station (MEPS) a few weeks later and stood in long lines with other would be recruits to have various medical tests performed on him. After being poked and stuck and palpated and otherwise violated by the civilian medical staff he was cleared for military service.

With his expectations and dreams in hand he entered the final step of his processing experience.

In an office on upper level of the MEPS station was an Army administrator who, unbeknownst to James, would decide his fate for the next five years. This was the first military person that James met who didn't smile or act particularly nice towards him. She was in her late twenties, maybe early thirties with cold eyes and a flat, but stern affect. "And your name is…" the sergeant requested. "I'm James Sanders, how are you?"

"Recruit Sanders, I'm going to get you assigned for training for your military occupational specialty in the Army. Your training will begin upon completion of basic training. Let's see what we have." She typed briefly on the computer to display a list of positions that the Army would like filled.

"I want to be a Predator pilot" James announced with pride and conviction. His imagination soared with his vision of the small aircraft as it rolls and glides on the wind, over the mountains and across vast terrain. James smiled and sat back in the rather hard chair.

"There aren't any openings for predator pilots. It looks like we have medical logistics, dispersing and payroll, combat mess specialist, and infantry. Which sounds good to you?"

Unfamiliar with the military nomenclature for occupational specialties and still stunned by his dream being so quickly and brutally dashed by this uncaring bureaucrat, James entered the fog of war for the first time. "Umm, I want to be a predator pilot." James' bottom lip poked out and his shoulders slumped.

James' sad look and one track mindedness touched the sergeant in a special place inside and she extended her nurturing support honed by years of military service. "Look, there ain't no dam pilot schools available right now! You've got to pick something else. If you want I can pick one for you." Scott was stunned by the harshness and paralyzed by the loss of his dream. "Look, recruit, a Predator school position might come open and you can apply for it later on. But for right now you've got to pick something else to get into. Ask your drill instructor about changing assignments when you get to basic. They can help you out." This last statement was perhaps the cruelest advice that James had ever received. But, with his hopes renewed he examined the list of jobs that were available in an attempt to find one that would look good on paper. At least till the occupational specialty was changed to "Predator Pilot". "So what do these positions do?" James inquired of the mean woman across the desk.

Without trying to conceal her irritation, the sergeant granted James a brief description. "Medical logistics handles medical supplies for the hospitals, and aid stations. Have you ever seen MASH?" James nodded. "Well they'll make sure units like that have the supplies they need." That didn't seem too bad, but not very exciting James thought. Seeing that he didn't bite on the first one the sergeant continued. "Dispersing and payroll make sure that other service members get paid properly and that their leave is calculated properly. They handle the service records and make sure other members can do their jobs, like the Predator pilots." The jab didn't go unnoticed by James. But spending his days pushing papers wasn't what he wanted to do during his military career. "Combat Mess Specialists prepare meals for troops in the field." James knew he didn't want to be a military cook. That position reeked of hard thankless work, long hours, and no excitement. "And the infantry, well, have you ever seen the movie Full Metal Jacket?" A flashback of mangled limbs and post-traumatic stress disorder was thrust into the front of James's mind. He shook his head no, declining that offer.

"Umm, I guess the medical logistics seems like it'll be ok." James conceded. "Good" the sergeant typed some more at her terminal. Eventually she printed a document and presented it to James who signed it, accepting the Army's terms of his surrender. For the next five years James would handle medical supplies for his country. He still dreamed of flying the Predator, but felt further from that position now than he was before he entered the wicked dream stealing witches office.

The enlisted oath was an interesting patriotic experience. It was like the Pledge of Allegiance on steroids to James, who raised his right hand along with the room full of other future service members. After the brief ceremony, the first of many during his military service, he palled around with the others for a while then eventually drove back home. Over the next several weeks James enjoyed a few outings with his friends and family. He packed his belongings in boxes and put them into the basement storage of his parent's house. This place where he grew up would no longer be his home. He wasn't sure what lay ahead for him after he got into the Army, but right now he was overwhelmed by mixed feelings of relief and sadness at leaving the only place he'd ever known.

***

Sandy also came to the health department by way of another career. This administrative assistant position was a dream come true when she received it. In contrast to the relative peace and stability of the health department, Sandy's home life growing up was difficult. As far back as she can remember her mother brought different men in and out of the house. She and her younger sister and brother would witness violence that should never been shown to children. Her mother would wear cuts and bruises so frequently that the condition was considered normal by the children by the time they were in middle school and high school. Sandy remembered one particularly bad night when the man her mother had been seeing for a couple of months came back to the home very late and drunk or high. Maybe he was both. Her mother wouldn't let him inside as he pounded on the door and cussed at her at the top of his lungs. Eventually Sandy's mother caved in, she always caved in. She went to the door, still wearing her night clothes and opened it. The despot struck her in the face with brass knuckles dislodging three teeth and splattering the wall and floor with her blood. He straddled her after she fell. He punched her repeatedly until her mother was an unresponsive bloody mess. The children huddled together atop the stairs viewing the carnage from between the railing posts unable to offer aid or even to speak lest the violence be directed towards them.

The man stood after completing his mauling and peered down at his victim. Realizing that he'd gone too far he stepped away from the unconscious woman. Maybe he heard the children, or perhaps felt their gaze on him because he lifted his head to view them. His expression, a cold, arrogant stare burned into the Sandy's mind for what seemed like hours. He then turned to face the door and departed never to be seen again.

A neighbor must have heard the commotion and called the police because they arrived a few moments after the villain escaped. When the officers arrived they called for the paramedics and began a search for her mother's attacker. They never found him. The paramedics came and put Sandy's mother on a stretcher. They started an IV and began bandaging her wounds, but the bandages became soaked with blood as quickly as the medics applied them. The children watched as an oxygen mask was placed on their mother's face and she was wheeled to the awaiting ambulance. They continued to huddle together.

A police officer climbed the stairs and approached them. Wide eyed the children observed the officer as he ascended the stairs towards their position. "Hey guys, my name is Officer Larry. Are any of you hurt?" His voice was soothing and confident. He knelt to approximate their level. The children shook their heads no. The officer observed the children looking for signs of injures, but didn't touch them out of respect. He knew through his training and experience that touching could be considered either comforting or threatening, and since he didn't know which he chose to use only his words. "Your mom is going to the hospital. The doctors there will take care of her. You'll be able to see her soon, but right now we need to take you somewhere safe." The words were reassuring to the scared children and they welcomed the pleasantries. "Can you follow me to my car so I can take you someplace safe?" the officer asked. Empowering the children with a choice was the best way to gain their confidence and aid the transition. He was still waiting for the location of the foster home where the children would reside, at least in the short term until they could either locate family members to take them, or their mother was released. The officer had seen enough assaults to know that it would be some time before the mother would recover enough to come home and care for the kids.

The children stood and followed the officer down the stairs. The youngest took the officer's hand. As the child grasped his hand he looked down and smiled a reassuring smile which gave a little comfort to them. The children followed Officer Larry through the main room of the home. Blood was pooled on the floor and splattered on the walls. Streaks of blood were drawn by the wheels of the gurney from where their mother laid to the front door. Officer Larry answered his radio. The call seemed to convey the location of the foster home where they would be taken. "Roger that." Officer

Larry said into his radio after receiving the address and name of the foster parents. He opened the back door to his police cruiser and helped the children in. They were buckled up. "Is this your first ride in a police car?" Officer Larry asked. The two youngest children gave him a blank stare while Sandy nodded her head in affirmation. The policeman closed the children's door and opened his own. He sat in the driver's seat and spoke again on the radio announcing that he was departing the home en route to the address provided.

The drive took about thirty minutes, but seemed longer. Street lights shown though the car windows, shimmered against the dark sky as they passed by the car at great speed. Officer Larry turned on the car radio to fill the still night with the sounds of familiar lyrics and melodies. Eventually, the car ride concluded at a home in a quiet neighborhood. Officer Larry parked the squad car at the front of the home that was well lit by a couple of porch lights and lanterns leading from the sidewalk up the walkway to the porch. Officer Larry opened the back door of the car and announced to the children "We are here." The tone was friendly and excited as if the children should expect a welcome surprise. Shortly after he opened the door to the car a couple exited the house and approached the awaiting children; who were themselves exiting the car near the officer. Still in their night clothes and robed for the cool night, Jim and his partner Mike greeted Officer Larry and then the children. "Hi there" Mike said to the kids. "My name is Mike, this is Jim. We are going to be taking care of you for a while." Mike lowered his height to closely match the children's as the officer had done earlier. "What are your names?" The children were silent; they only looked at the gentlemen overwhelmed, scared, tired, and hungry. Mike stood and held Jim's hand. "Come on inside, we have dinner for you and beds made when you're ready." Sandy looked at the officer and he smiled and nodded. He followed the children to the house and left them at the door. Speaking to the oldest, Officer Larry gave her a piece of paper with his name and phone number. "If you need something call me. These are good people and they'll take care of all of you till your mom gets better." With that the policeman shook hands with Mike and Jim and bid them good night before returning to his car.

The inside of the house was warm and comfortable. The home smelled like beef stew. The ample lighting illuminated the large home revealing the plush furnishings, and cozy décor. The children passed through the foyer and through a living room to the large dining room near the kitchen. They each sat at a large chair and were soon joined by Mike and Jim. "Do you like soup?" Jim inquired of the kids. Famished, the youngest gripped the spoon aside his bowl in eager anticipation of sustenance. Mike served the soup to the kids. It was delicious. They ate seconds, and then thirds. Mike and Jim, who had eaten earlier, watched the children devour the servings. They knew only a little about the terrors the night had brought the young ones, but they would do all they could to nurture them and keep them safe in the coming weeks. Their home was a waypoint for children who had fallen on hard times, but those children were all made better by passing through.

***

Scott completes his morning greeting with the administrative staff and stops by his office. He turns on his computer and sets his bag next to his desk. The investigator Retrieves his ancient coffee cup he received from the National Sexually Transmitted Disease Conference in Denver Colorado, which is also printed on the cup for posterity reasons, from its resting place on his desk and leaves for the employee lounge. Scott and his trusty cup make their way through the main floor of the building and up the stairs located behind the laboratory. The aroma of fresh brewed coffee drifts down the stairwell. Following the heavenly scent of coffee, Scott arrives at the employee lounge. There he finds not only the sought after beverage, but also Nurse Marge who is sitting at the lounge table enjoying some oatmeal and coffee herself. "Morning Marge" Scott greets the middle aged woman in blue and white scrubs with flowers printed on the top. "Good morning Scott, thank God it's Friday." Black framed glasses dominate the face of the otherwise visually unremarkable woman. She wears a simple smooth gold wedding band and silver watch on her left hand. Small gold crosses dangle lightly from her earlobes and a simple gold pendent is suspended around her neck. She has ear buds inserted into both ears, but the volume is low enough for her to monitor what is going on around her. Scott can't hear what she's listening to, but imagines it is early morning religious programming.

Scott briskly walks to the counter where the coffee pot is housed. There is a variety of disposable paper cups, a container of disposable stirs, and several containers of powered creamer, sugar packets, and sweeteners surrounding the coffee pot. It is as if the appliance is enshrined in the room. Scott uses the French vanilla powered creamer and adds a sweetener packet to the cup before pouring the coffee. The ingredients mix well by the time the cup is filled requiring a minimum amount of stirring. Scott samples the creation and affirms its goodness with an audible "Mmmm."

Marge is reading actively on her E reader while finishing her breakfast. That's not surprising because the health department nurse is usually reading something when not actively engaged in providing patient care. This morning she is reading a New article about a new study linking religious affiliation with divorce. She views the small device with great focus as if hanging on each word. Marge's ability to multitask is impressive to Scott. He thinks to himself "I find it difficult to walk and chew gum at the same time. This nurse is eating, listening to something, reading, and conversing with me. Wow." Aloud to the nurse, Scott says "Well Marge, enjoy your morning, I'll see you again soon I'm sure." Scott salutes with his cup and prepares to go back to work. "You too Scott" she lifts her head from the e- reader. "Have a blessed day."

Scott descends the steps and passes Ann on the way. She is wearing a red business suit with a knee length skirt and matching heals. In her arms are an overcoat, brief case, and a manila folder she must have picked up at the front desk on her way in. The folder probably contains some faxes that came in while the clinic was closed. "How's your morning so far Ann?"

"Busy as usual. I have three days' worth of work to finish today before the weekend, including this grant." Ann holds up the folder as evidence of her excessive workload. "Oh" Scott sympathizes, "the main thing is the keep the main thing the main thing I suppose." The phrase takes a couple of seconds to register for an already stressed brain but Ann appreciates the advice. "Thanks, I'll keep that in mind." She climbs the steps with determination while Scott walks down towards his office.

When he arrives he finds Sara standing outside his office holding a tablet and pen. "Good morning Sara, how was your evening?" "It was fine Scott, how was yours?" After the initial pleasantries the two enter the small room and have a seat. "So what questions do you have about yesterday?" Scott begins the work discussion with an excellent open ended question.

"I'm just taking it all in right now. It's a lot of new information to process." Sara has been studying the basic training classes from the Centers for Disease Control over the week and is only half finished. The self paced computer classes give new disease investigators an in-depth education concerning anatomy, disease characteristics, and the basics of field investigations. Scott recalls going through the training himself, though it was through correspondence courses back then. It really is a lot of information to learn and apply. But, it is necessary for them to be considered subject matter experts. The reality is that after all of the training it will still take a full year for Sara to be a completely competent disease investigator.

"How far along are you?" Scott sits back in his chair. "I've finished seven of the fifteen modules." Sara replies with a muted enthusiasm. Her expectation was that she would easily and quickly complete these courses, especially after the rigors of graduate school.

"Ok" Scott accepts the progress report "well, see what you can get done this morning and I'll come get you if anything interesting comes up." Nodding, Sarah leaves Scott's office for her own.

It doesn't take long for something interesting to come up. James comes by Scott's office carrying a large envelope delivered a few moments earlier. "Hey Scott, mail came and the labs are here. Do you want them or do you want me to give them to nurse Marge?"

"I'll take them James, Thanks."

James hands Scott the envelope and returns to the front desk. Scott opens the envelope and begins to go through the stack of laboratory test results. The majority of them are negative results from routine screenings. Women who were tested at their annual well woman exams, the maternal and infant care clinic's screening for pregnant women, and tests from the STD clinic are all contained in this package. Scott sees several positive Chlamydia tests, a few Gonorrhea test, a couple have both, and…a reactive Syphilis test on the woman he interviewed yesterday. Rose's Syphilis screening test came back highly reactive. The confirmation test is still pending, but with the Gonorrhea test also positive the chances that this is a false positive is slim. Scott puts the lab to the side and locates the her number. He dials it, but reaches a machine.

"Hi, you've reached Rose, I can't come to the phone right now, but leave your message after the beep and I might call you back."

"Hello Rose, this is Scott, we talked last night. I really need to talk with you again. Please call me as soon as you get this." Scott leaves his number on the voice mail.

The three guys she named during the Gonorrhea interview, Pritchard, Dustin, and Red, will all need to be tested and treated for Syphilis as well. It's a good thing he was able to talk with her yesterday. Finding syphilis early is crucial to stopping the spread. Given even a few days, Syphilis can spread like a wild fire and infect a lot of people. That endangers lives, but also makes it difficult to manage the outbreak. Finding these three guys is now a top priority.

Scott walks down to Sara's office. She is still settling in. The walls are bare and the book shelves are empty save a few technical manuals and old reference books. On her desk are the computer, printer, and a few pens. "Sara, do you remember that woman Rose we talked with yesterday afternoon?"

"Yes, she was the last one with gonorrhea, with the three partners."

"Good memory, well her Syphilis test came back positive. Those three partners will need to be located, tested, and treated."

"Was she treated yet?" Sara inquires?

"Not yet" Scott applauding her for paying attention. "I just called her, but haven't heard back yet. We'll get her in for additional testing, treatment, and can talk with her again."

"Don't we have everything we need already?" Sara says referring to the interview from the previous day.

"She was interviewed for Gonorrhea. The time lines are different for Syphilis. Also we talk with people who have syphilis and HIV more than once. It gives us the opportunity to be more thorough. It also gives the patient some time to think about the interview process. They often give us additional partners during the second and third interviews."

"OK, so what are we going to do?"

"Plan to go back to the field this afternoon. We need to find Rose's partners Dustin and Pritchard. I'll look up their info this morning and be ready to go soon after." Scott says. Sara receives the news of working with patients very well. She's been in school for a long time and is ready to get her feet wet. Even if this isn't the pool she would have selected.

"Sounds good" Sara says with renewed energy. She returns to her CDC online training determined to learn the specifics of this position. Though, the thought of reading an endless stream of computer screens about Syphilis isn't very appealing. "I'll be in my office, reading, if you need me." Scott excuses himself and walks down the hall towards his office.

The name "Pritchard Wallace" is typed into the data base in an attempt to locate the exposed man's where a bouts. "There he is." Scott exclaims as a match is found. The address and phone number are old. Pritchard must have received immunizations as a child there at the clinic. Still, the address is listed and likely belonged to either his parents or other close family members. It's a good place to start. Scott writes down the locating information on a tablet near his keyboard. He tries the phone number first. "Hello?" a woman's voice comes over the receiver. "Hi, my name is Scott and I need to talk with Pritchard Wallace." The woman tells Scott, "There's no one by that name here." Scott, realizing it was a long shot concludes the conversation. "Thank you, I'm sorry to have bothered you." The line goes dead. Few people keep a phone number for very long, and several years was a lot to hope for, but still, sometimes an investigator can get lucky. Scott prepares a referral letter and envelope for this afternoon's visit to the address and affixes it to the clip board.

He next types in the name Dustin Evens in to the search section of the clinic's data base. A record is found with the latest entry being a few months ago. Scott notes that this patient was seen because he was exposed to Chlamydia at that time and was treated but not tested. That's not uncommon. Guys don't like to get "swabbed." "Swabbed" is an apt term for the collection method used to detect Gonorrhea and Chlamydia. A small cue tip like probe is inserted into the guy's urethra in hopes of getting some of the bacteria on the tip. That sample is then sent to the laboratory for analysis. While the test collection is uncomfortable, it's no where near as painful as some patients fear or their responses would indicate. The test itself is very good at determining whether or not a person is infected. That is to say that the test is both sensitive and specific.

***

Sara props her head on her hands while she reads, "Sensitivity verses Specificity" The module continues regarding laboratory tests. "Good, this is one that was covered well in graduate school." Sara again enjoys the overlap between her formal education and her disease investigator training. If a person has a disease the test should be positive (sensitivity). If a person doesn't have a disease the test should read negative (specificity). The test reads "Basically, Sensitivity is how well a test detects the disease. The more sensitive the test, the more likely it will identify the presence of disease. While specificity describes how reliable the test is at detecting the absence of disease. The more specific the test the more accurately it will tell someone who is not infected that they are truly not infected." The module continues "Let's say there are 100 people in a population where we know for a fact that half of the people are infected with a disease. A highly sensitive test will identify 50 people who are infected. While a test that is not as sensitive may find 60 or 40 people in the same population. It's just not as accurate. The opposite is true of specificity. A test that is very specific will tell us that fifty people do not have the disease. This is important for a couple of reasons. First, all lab tests have some inherent error. Also, this points out the reason screening tests are supported with confirmation tests because one is very sensitive while the other is very specific.

***

Scott writes down the phone number and address for Dustin Evens on the same pad. He lifts the receiver and dials the number. A faded poor quality recording of a popular rap song plays for ninety seconds before a man's voice, presumably Dustin's, comes on. "Yo this is Big D, you know what to do." Refraining from calling the patient "Big D," Scott leaves a professional message "This message is for Dustin Evens, My name is Scott and I have important health information for you. Please call me at…" The message is short on details, but the reasoning for that is to protect Dustin's confidentiality in case someone else hears his messages. Scott prepares another referral with Dustin's address and places that with the other on the clip board.

His phone rings. "This is Scott." Nurse Peggy is on the other line. "Scott, I've got one for you to look at." "Be right there Peggy." Scott grabs a tablet, his pen, and a stack of picture cards and leaves his office to meet with the clinic nurse and a patient in the exam room. Scott reaches Examination Room # 2 and knocks on the door. "Come in" he hears Peggy say from inside. Upon opening the door he sees James Jefferson, the teen from last night. "Hi James, what's going on?" Scott inquires after closing the door behind him. "It looks like Mr. Jefferson has a sore on his penis" the clinic nurse brings Scott up to speed on the findings. "How long have you had this James?" Scott says as he puts on polyurethane gloves that are perhaps a little too small. "I just noticed it" the scared teen states with conviction. "Let me take a look at it," Scott requests of the boy. He stands and unfastens his pants and pulls them down exposing his penis to the medical staff. Scott examines the dime sized sore with raised edges that appears to be resolving. "Does it hurt or itch?" Scott asks. "No, it's just there. Doesn't bother me. I just came in cause you said I needed to get a shot for that Gonorrhea thing." The nurse found the lesion while conducting an examination, and a very good thing she did. "That looks like a syphilis lesion James. How long have you had it again?" "I told you I just saw it" he states again, this time with even more conviction. "Yes, you did, but I need to know how long you've really had this." The challenge from Scott to his assertion comes as a surprise to the boy. "This lesion is healing, that means it's been here for a while." Looking down, the young man confesses, "It's been a couple of weeks." "Ok" Scott says, "Well we are going to get some blood from you and go ahead and treat you for Syphilis. What do you know about Syphilis, James?" "Ain't that what got Capone?" he answers. Scott, mildly impressed by the patient's historical knowledge of the disease goes on "Him and a whole lot of other people before penicillin was discovered and widely used.

Syphilis is a disease that is caused by bacteria. You got it by having sex with someone who has it. If it goes untreated it can lead to some really dangerous health problems. Basically it can maim people, make them crazy, and then kill them." While the description of this disease is shocking, it's also brutally honest. Scott is preparing James for the imminent interview. Scott washes his hands and encourages the patient to do the same. He picks up the receiver from the wall mounted phone and calls Sara's office. "Health department, this is Sara." "Hey Sara, this is Scott, can you come to exam room # 2 please?" "Be right there" Sara hangs up the receiver and vacates her office for the patient care area. She arrives at exam room # 2 and knocks lightly on the door. "Who is it?" Scott responds from inside. Nurse Peggy cuts her eyes at Scott tilting her head and puckering her lips as if to suggest the questioning is unnecessary. "It's Sara" the voice is a little stressed and very polite. Scott, lifting his palms to his chest as if to say "What?" to the clinic nurse, calls back to Sara, "Come in." She opens the door and enters the room, paper and pen in hand. She closes the door behind her. "James, this is my partner Sara." "Hi James" Sara recognizes the young man from last night. "What up," the patient reciprocates with a head nod. "James, can you show Sara the sore?" He sighs and stands, revealing himself again to the room of medical personnel, this time more embarrassed due to the presence of an attractive younger woman. "Have you ever seen one of these" Scott inquires of Sara. "Just in the texts." Sara observes the lesion.

"Here you go." Scott hands Sara the box of gloves. Sara, with a slightly disgusted expression, takes the box and selects two gloves from within. She applies them and takes the patient's penis into her hands. "Feel the borders of the lesion" Scott advises. She complies. They are raised and hard. James doesn't react when the wound is touched telling her that it is painless. She releases the penis and removes the gloves, immediately washing her hands with a copious amount of soap. Scott advises the teenager to wash his hands again. "That sore is highly infectious, even if it doesn't hurt. You need to make sure you wash your hands well after touching it." Understanding Scott's point, James nods in agreement. "We are going to step out while Nurse Peggy gets you taken care of. We'll talk some more before you leave though. Peggy, can you let me know when you're done, please?" Peggy, who is already preparing the injections on the counter, responds without looking at Scott, "You know I will." Scott and Sara exit the room and walk towards Scott's office. "Ok young man, one more time. I need you to drop your trousers. These are going into your hips." She holds up two syringes of benzathine penicillin G, a white viscous medication affixed to two long needles. The well prodded patient sighs, shakes his head and stands. He again undoes his pants and shows the nurse his butt cheeks. He lifts his shirt and bends over the exam table. The nurse wipes one cheek with an alcohol prep pad. The pad is cool and wet, but the anticipation of the pain dominates the young man's mind. "Ok, little poke in three...two..."

"Ahhhhh!" He responds to the injection as the thick medication is slowly pushed into his butt muscle. "Ok, one more." The nurse places the syringe into a nearby red plastic box attached to the wall. James winces as he lifts his shirt to clear the way for the other injection. "Ok, Three…Two…"

After the two penicillin shots the old nurse has the patient pull his pants up and take a seat on the exam table. She then rolls up his sleeve and approaches him with yet another injection. "What's that for?!" he responds with vibrant objection. "This is for the Gonorrhea sweetie." She smiles. The boy slumps, he'd forgotten about that. "Three…two…" "Ouch! This sucks." The nurse places a band aid over the injection site and consoles the boy with a rub on his shoulder. "Just got to take these pills and you're all done." "What are the pills for" he inquires, feeling as though he'd received enough treatment for the day. "It's to help with the shot to take care of the Gonorrhea." "The gonorrhea that I don't even think I have?" he states in a half question half accusation. "Yes dear" the nurse hands him two paper cups. One has water in it and the other four small pink pills. "Gonorrhea is a tricky little bugger. It changes so that medications don't work on it any more. We have to give you a shot and pills now to get rid of it. Have you eaten recently." "No one told me I needed to eat. Why, does that matter?" James asks, clearly frustrated at this point. "Well, the pills may make you feel a little sick, like you have food poisoning for a few hours." "Great!" James expresses his frustration with sarcasm. The old nurse opens a drawer in the cabinet and gets out a juice box and a small package of crackers. "Here, eat this. It should make you feel better." The boy opens the juice box and the package of crackers. His bottom is getting sore and he's tired of being at the clinic.

"When Peggy is done treating James, we'll bring him back to the office for the interview. That way she can use the room for other patients. Also, bringing him back here is a little more comfortable place for us to talk. When I talk with the patient I ask that you don't say anything during the interview. Just observe. Any questions you have just write them down and we'll address them later. You've already learned some of the do's and don'ts of interviewing. Here are some things you won't read in the manuals: For starters, patients lie about sex, symptoms, partners, and just about anything else you can think of. Secondly, everyone is hiding something."

"That seems cynical. Are you sure you haven't done this job too long?" Sara retorts. "Well, those aren't my rules, Sara, they were taught to me by my mentor Mike Epps years ago. I've found that the rules can be applied and assumed to be literally true for almost every investigation. But the principle is what's important. What it means is that we must keep digging until we get nothing more from the patient. They are hiding some critically important piece of information that we could use to save someone's life. You haven't been to the retirement home and seen people suffering from dementia caused by neurosyphilis yet, but you will. And you'll want to prevent that from happening to other people if you care about what you do. I'll push patients to give me what I need to save lives, and yes that makes them uncomfortable, angry even. But in the end I'm doing it because I care."

The phone rings again, "Scott?" "Yes Peggy." "He's ready for you now."

"OK, I'll be right there." Scott hangs up the phone. "Now this guy is going to lie, but we need to know who he's had sex with." He leaves the room to escort the patient back to the office.

"Hey James, how were the shots?" Scott inquires as he comes in the treatment room. "Man, that shit sucked!" a disgruntled James expresses his dissatisfaction with Scott. "Ya, those are some nasty shots. The stuff is pretty thick. You're going to want to do some walking around to help absorb it. A heating pad might help too." Scott advises James. "Follow me, we are going to go to my office to talk." "What's there to talk about, I'm taken care of now?" The boy asks. "I don't want to talk in the hall, it's not private. We'll discuss it more in my office." The two walk down the hall and go into Scott's office.

"Do you have any questions about Syphilis James?" Scott sits at his desk, the boy in a chair on the side of it. "Naw, you already told me."

"Ok, well part of what I do is get in contact with other people who may have been exposed so that we can get them tested and treated too. It's crucial that we don't let people get sick and/or die from this infection. Also, everything we talk about is completely confidential. I don't tell anyone outside this clinic what we've talked about, and even then, only if they need to know. Now I have some cards that I want you to take a look at. There are pictures of syphilis symptoms on the cards. Just tell me if you or any of your partners have had anything that looks like the pictures." Scott removes the rubber band that is holding the cards together and shows James the first card. It is a picture of a sore like the one James has on his penis. "That looks like what I got." James recognizes the lesion. Scott continues his education "This is a syphilis chancre, also called a primary lesion. It appears three weeks after you get infected. The good thing about syphilis is that since it's predictable we can actually tell who gave it to whom. Have you seen anything like this on any of your partners?" Scott asks about partners, plural, because it creates the assumption that the patient has more than one making it easier for him to admit to multiple sex partners. People will usually meet expectation. "No, just the one on me" James states. "OK," Scott moves onto the next card that shows a pair of arms with spots on them and the palms. "Have you seen anything like this on your partners? It's a secondary symptom of syphilis that usually shows up a few weeks after the lesion goes away. The rash on the palms of the hands and soles of the feet are classic syphilis symptoms." The young man looks at the picture and the wheels turn. He pauses for a moment then answers. "I aint had sex with nobody with that on them." Scott, sensing that he has more information on the matter rephrases the question. "Have you seen anything like this on any of your friends? Remember, this disease can kill people. Telling me could save their life." James looks at the floor, but Scott continues. "Remember, I don't tell them anything about you. Just like how I came and talked with you about the Gonorrhea. Did I tell you anything about who told me you'd been exposed?" James shakes his head. "Right, and I won't tell them anything about you either."

"Alright man, I seen that rash on the hands. This dude named Grimy had it a couple weeks back." Scott takes his pad and writes the information down that the patient is telling him. "What's Grimy's real name?" Scott asks. "Man, I don't know that. Just goes by Grimy." Scott concedes, "Where's Grimy staying?"

Lifting his eyes from the floor and watching the paper James describes the house to the best of his abilities. Scott writes down the directions and the description of the house with as much detail as he can gather from the young man's memory. "So when's the last time you had sex with Grimy?" The young man looked offended by the question. "Man I don't do no dudes!" Scott motions with his hand for him to relax. "OK, I'm not judging you. Some men have sex with other men and that's ok, we just need to know who all's been exposed."

"Who is the last person you had sex with?"

"Just some bitch I met at a party." James is uncooperative again.

"What party did you meet her at?" Scott follows up.

"We hooked up at Grimy's place."

Grimy. What Scott wouldn't give for a chance to test and interview this guy. Grimy is a possible core transmitter, meaning that he is an efficient spreader for sexually transmitted disease. Finding him could be key to disease abatement in this community.

"What's her first name?"

"Angela, I don't know her last name."

Scott writes down the woman's first name. He didn't get lucky enough to have an unusual name that he could search for in the data base, but there are many ways to find people. "What does Angela look like?"

"She's 5'5, nice hips, big titties..."

James goes on to describe Angela in as much detail as he can including a tattoo of paw prints leading up one of her thighs. "When did you have sex with Angela?" Scott uses the woman's name instead of a third person identifier to encourage the patient to think of her as a person, someone who is in danger and needs help.

"It's been a couple weeks."

"When's the first time you had sex with her?"

"It was just that time."

This new information concerns Scott greatly because of the source spread relationship. Every person who is infected gets the infection from someone else. That person who infected James is his "source". James may have had sex with Angela while he had the highly infections lesion. And if he infected her she would be a "spread" from James. Scott's primary role in the health department is identifying source spread candidates. Scott's identified a possible spread, but James was infected by someone else.

"Who did you have sex with before Angela?

He names Tiffany and Regan. Both are classmates in high school. Scott gets all of the information about these two young ladies from James and writes them down. James claims he last had sex with them about 2 months ago, but he used condoms.

"So who else?"

"That's it."

Scott talks to James some more. He gets more information about his demographic information, drug use history, and a couple of friends who James doesn't have sex with, but should be tested anyway.

"Well James, thank you for all of your help. Do you have any questions?"

"No, I just wana leave."

Scott smiles "well you're free to go. I'll need to meet with you again later. I'll call you when we get your test results back." James gets up and stiffly walks out of the office to the clinic entrance. He rubs his right butt cheek as he limps down the hall.

"So what do you think?" Scott turns to Sara.

"I think we've got a problem at that high school." Sara presents her assessment.

"He didn't get syphilis from Tiffany or Regan."

"What do you mean? Those are the only other people he named who could have given it to him." Sara asserts.

"Syphilis travels in social networks among people who have a lot of sex. These two girls don't fit into the demographics, social determinants. For starters they are too young. Their biggest risk for syphilis is having sex with James, but he didn't have a lesion while having sex with them so they won't be spread candidates." James notices that Sara appears doubtful. "Don't get me wrong, we are still going to find them and test them, but there's someone else."

"What questions do you have?"

"Why were you asking about his friends, the one's he's not having sex with?"

"Good questions. It's called clustering. Because disease spreads in social networks like friends, golf buddies, crack addicts, and so on and so forth, it's important to know who these people are. James had sex with someone with Syphilis. It makes sense that his friends may have similar risks. Maybe they even had sex with the same source. Also, it gives James an out. If he has a partner that, for whatever reason, he doesn't want to tell us about he can call them a "friend" and we'll still get them tested. More information is always better."

"So how are you going to find out who infected him?"

Scott raises his eyebrows "That's the million dollar question. Right now what we have are leads. We'll talk to Tiffany and Regan. They might know more about who James is having sex with, if they exist. Another possibility is that James may call me and tell me about the person he "forgot about". Yet another possibility is that James may go tell the other person or people that they need to get tested. In which case, they'll probably show up here or at the hospital emergency room. They'll tell us that he referred them and we can make the connection that way. If none of that works out there are still some other things we can do. We don't have any open Syphilis cases right now making James our index patient. This investigation has just started."

Sara knows from school that the index patient is the first patient found with the disease. She also realizes the elephant in the room. "Scott?"

"Ya, what's up?" Scott looks up from his notes at the young investigator.

"Who named him in the Gonorrhea investigation that got him to come to the clinic in the first place?"

Scott nods, thinking to himself that she'll work out just fine. "Peaches. She was tested last week, but we are still pending results for the syphilis test."

"Why didn't he tell us about her?" Sara is a little taken aback.

"We don't know yet, but it gives us something else to talk to him about. I couldn't ask him about Peaches without indicating that she named him. That would violate her confidentiality. But I'm not going to let it go either. If he doesn't name her back then we know there are other partners somewhere out there."

"I think he's using crack." Sara points out.

"Why do you say that?" Scott replies.

"That guy Grimy is a crack dealer and it seems obvious that if James is going to parties at Grimy's house he's also using drugs with him."

"But he denied drug use." Scott points out.

Sara smiles and nods "He lied."

Chapter 4

Getting a location for Grimy house is the biggest payoff for this investigation so far. And Scott means to cash in that check now. "Grab your stuff, we're going to see Grimy." Sara stands and gathers her few belongings from Scott's office and leaves. She quickly passes down the hall where she meets Ann going to opposite way. "Hi Sara, how is the training coming along?"

Sara, clearly excited by her expression and hurried manor tells the boss "Great, we've got a Syphilis case and now we are going to try to make contact with some people who might be exposed."

"Alright…that's good I suppose." The administrator has mixed feelings about describing the discovery of a Syphilis case as "good," but she's understands why this would be exciting to the new investigator. "Good luck."

"Thanks." Sara's response is short and enthusiastic as her focus is solely on the upcoming field trip to the crack dealer's house. She quickly gathers her coat, a soft shell brief case, a pad of paper, and a couple of pens from her desk. She turns off the light in her office and briskly walks back to Scott's towards the front of the clinic.

While Sara was away Scott used Google maps to identify the location of Grimy's crack house. There was even a picture of it. Didn't look like a crack house from the picture, but the best ones don't. Scott printed the map and put together a referral. The outside of the envelope only reads "Grimy." Scott wishes he had a real name, but works with what he has. He retrieves his coat from the hook attached to his office door and grabs his bag from beside his desk. He also gets a soft shell nylon cooler from his filing cabinet. This bag, which looks as if it should carry his lunch, is Scott's blood kit. It has everything he needs to draw blood in the field and has been with him since he started. He opens the bag and checks the dates on the blood tubes. "Good, they haven't expired yet." He inventories the rest of the contents. In the bag he finds alcohol pads, vacationers, needles, tourniquets, cotton balls, band aids, and a container with absorbing material inside for the specimens.

His rib starts to bother him again and Scott sits for a moment. He's glad to have a good lead. He's also glad that Sara is catching on to the job quickly. But he feels like someone pulled his battery out. "I just need a minute. Maybe a little more coffee" he tells himself. By this time the coffee which held so much joy for him a couple hours earlier is now lukewarm. Still, it's better than nothing so Scott takes a few large gulps of the now cold coffee.

"Ready?!" the overly perky voice meets Scott's defused motivation.

"Ya, let's go."

The investigators arrive at the address a few moments later. It's not far from the clinic and was thankfully easy to find. The house, a two story yellow split level with a large front yard is situated between two well maintained homes in a decent neighborhood. There's no fence or front porch and the yard has patches of missing grass. The windows are all covered with blinds and a remote security camera is barely visible from the street. "OK, be careful as we approach." Scott advises his protégé. "Drug dealers have been known to keep vicious dogs on the roof of their houses. When the police or other unwanted visitors arrive the dogs leap down on top of the intruders and maul them." Sara's expression is a mix between horror and disbelief. She doesn't know if she should take the veteran seriously, but she takes a long look at the roof of the house out of reflex. Scott chuckles.

They approach the front door and Scott knocks. Sara looks up searching for vicious dogs. "Who is it?!" a stern voice booms from within. "I'm Scott, looking for Grimy."

"What do you want?!" The angry voice replies. In Scott's mind this is a big win. The guy inside didn't deny the existence of the person he was looking for which was a big concern when he came out here. Especially given the difficulty finding this guy in the past. "I need to talk with him about an important health matter." The phrase is vague and well rehearsed.

The door opens. A short skinny man, about 5'3 stands before them. He's wearing a stained whitish wife beater and shorts that come down to his mid calf. Shower shoes and socks cover the man's feet. His face is scarred and pitted and his lips are crusted with white flakes that may be dry skin or drool. "Who the fuck are you?"

"My name is Scott, this is my co worker Sara. Are you Grimy?" The pun was not intended, but the irony hits Scott like an epiphany. He maintains his composure. Sara smiles at the man "Hi."

"Ya, what you want?"

"We are with the health department and came out here to tell you that you may have been exposed to Syphilis." Scott pauses for a moment to allow the words to sink in for the man.

"Man, I aint got no Syph a shit."

"Well we can do some testing for you, just to make sure you're OK. Can we come in?" Sara shoots Scott a look that he catches out of the corner of his eye. Her enthusiasm may be dampened some by her sense of self preservation. Grimy motions for the two to come in and Scott follows with Sara closely behind.

The house smells like body odor, trash that needs to be taken out, and cat urine. The powerful stench is matched only by its filth. The front door opens into the living room that has a couple of couches, lazy boy style chairs, a large coffee table, and an entertainment center with a large flat screen TV. Dirty dishes clutter the top of the coffee table, and full trash bags rest peacefully against the far wall buzzing from the sound of flies. "Have a seat," Grimy points to a vacant couch near the chair where he just plopped down. Scott thinks the couch was at some point cream colored, but has evolved into a yellow with dark brown patches. "Thanks." Scott sits on the couch. Sara looks on in horror. "I'll stand" she declines the offer and folds her arms across her chest.

Scott removes a pad and pen from his bag. "I brought my blood kit so I can get some blood from you. I just have some forms for you to fill out so that we can run the test." Scott hands Grimy a couple of pieces of paper and a clip board. The forms are a registration form for the clinic, and a consent form for the testing. "Now this testing won't cost you anything and we should have your results back in a one to two weeks."

"What happens if I've got this?" Grimy's tone softens considerably from the initial contact.

Scott reassures the man, "We'll give you some shots that'll get rid of the syphilis. Now we are also going to do a test for HIV along with this." Grimy pauses for a moment upon hearing about the HIV test, but continues writing without question.

Scott puts on his gloves and sets up his test kit. When Grimy finishes filling out the forms he hands the clip board back to Scott who looks it over. "His name is Lawrence Polk, interesting." Scott says to himself. Scott didn't ask the man what his real name was because he didn't want to prompt him to lie. He also didn't want to admit that he didn't know his name thereby undermining his credibility.

"Which arm would you like?" Scott holds up the tourniquet and points at the Grimy's arms.

"This one I guess." Lawrence holds out his left arm. As he does Scott notices a splotchy rash on the man's arms. "How long have you had this rash?" Lawrence looks at it opening his hands and revealing a dark rash on both of his palms. "I don't know, like a week?"

Scott applies the tourniquet and finds a fat juice vein that protrudes beautifully from the inside of the patient's elbow. Scott pokes the vein with the needle and pushes the tub into the vacationer. Instantly the tube begins to fill with blood. After the receptacle is full, Scott removes the tube setting it to the side. He places the cotton ball over the needle and withdraws it from the vein while removing the tourniquet. "Hold pressure there." Scott motions to the cotton ball. He then opens a band aid and sticks it to the man's arm.

"That rash looks like it could be from Syphilis. "I'd like for you to come to the clinic so we can get you treated."

"Can't I just wait till my test results come back?"

"You can, but you don't want to have syphilis any longer than necessary. I can get you treated right now."

Just then a young woman walks down the steps. She has her hair up in a high pony tail and is wearing a baggy yellow t shirt with Sponge Bobs face printed on the front and short jean shorts. The jean shorts show off her tattoo of paw prints going up her left thigh. "Hey Grimy, what's going on?" she inquires regarding the unusual company.

"Noth'n bitch. Mind yo own." Lawrence replies in a defensive tone.

"I'm serious, what's going on." To her credit, she doesn't back down. Her assertiveness encourages Lawrence to inform her of the situation.

"They think I got Syphilis." Lawrence confesses. The woman becomes agitated and vocal.

"What? When were you going to tell me?! I knew I shouldn't have been mess'n with you!"

"Look bitch, I just found out. They can test you too."

Scott, recognizing the woman from James' description interjects. "Yes we can. If you can just fill out this form, miss, we can get started." Scott wants to get both of these two into the clinic today. But he doesn't want to overplay his hand. He gets a sample from her and she completes the registration form giving him her name, address, and number. "Can you two accompany me to the clinic and we'll get you treated?" The couple reluctantly agrees.

"I got to finish gett'n ready." Angela announces. She walks back upstairs and a door is heard shutting. Lawrence goes to a side room and comes back with a heavy black hooded coat, still wearing the capris for men and shower shoes with socks.

Scott teases Sara, "This might be a minute, are you sure you don't want to have a seat?" He only receives a cold look in response. Scott goes over some of his paperwork but feels something crawling on his ankle. Glancing down he sees a roach scurrying across his exposed flesh. Scott wipes the insect from his leg and stands. He picks up his bag from the floor where he placed it beside his legs. Whispering to Sara "We may need to shake out our stuff before we go home. Don't want any stowaways." Sara strongly dislikes the idea of bringing roaches back to her apartment and feels a little sick to her stomach.

After a few moments Angela comes back downstairs. This time she is in full length jeans and a coat with white fur around the border of the hood. "I'm ready" she announces to the three who are patiently waiting for her return. Lawrence opens the door and the four of them leave the house. Sara and Scott are happy to be outside breathing clean air, though their clothes have absorbed the stench of Lawrence's house. They walk over to Scott's car as he unlocks the doors with the remote. Sara sits in the front and Angela right behind her. Lawrence sits behind Scott. The ride is a little uncomfortable for the rear seat passengers since Scott's economy car doesn't accommodate four people very well. "The clinic isn't very far." Scott reassures the passengers.

Angela announces, "I've been there. It's by the Mexican food place." Lawrence looks at her and she continues "What?" Looking away Lawrence responds, "Noth'n." The rest of the ride to the clinic is quiet. Scott thinks about all of the things he wants to talk with them about. He makes a mental list and goes over the conversations in his mind. Sara wants to go by her apartment and put her clothes in the laundry and scrub every square inch of herself. Her legs and hair itch, but she's pretty sure it's psychosomatic.

They arrive at the clinic and park. Scott talks to the couple as they approach the main entrance. "I'm going to have both of you check in. You won't need to fill out a lot of paperwork because you've already done that when I drew your blood. They'll make a chart for you and then the nurse will call you back. I'll talk with both of you individually before I take you home. Any questions?"

"How long's this gona take?" Angela asks as if she has something more important to do.

"About thirty minutes to an hour give or take." Scott replies.

The front desk is busy with James and Sandy helping patients. "What's up, Scott?" James greets him after they walk in. "How's it going Sara?"

"James, can you get these two checked in? Here's their paperwork."

"Sure thing. Can you two please have a seat; we'll call you back shortly." James points to the waiting area and the couple finds two unoccupied seats fairly close together.

"Thanks James." Scott walks towards the exam rooms to find a nurse while Sara stops at the reception desk.

"What did I miss?" Sara asks James.

"Nothing exciting. About half of the people who've made appointments showed up. That's typical. Then we've had some walk ins with the usual complaints. How was the field?"

Sara laughed and scratched her head again. "It was ... educational."

Sandy listens in to the conversation while building the two charts and entering the patient information into the clinic's computer system. She looks at Lawrence with disdain, not caring for him at all. He reminds her of a childhood experience. She works hard to maintain her professionalism and to perform her duties to the high standard she is known for at the clinic. But his presence is an unmistakable distraction.

Sara leaves the reception desk and walks back to Scott's office. She looks in the open door and sees his head is on his desk. "You don't look so good. Maybe you should go home."

"I'm alright, just tired. Are they getting checked in?"

"Yes, the charts are almost completed."

"Can you tell Peggy or Marge that we brought in a couple of patients that need to be treated, please?" Scott looks up at Sara. He does look tired.

"Ya, of course. Anything else?" Sara is surprised. This is the first assignment that Scott's given her. He's been very hands on with everything and she's only been asked to observe. "I'll be right back."

"Thanks Sara" Scott calls after her. He takes another swallow of cold coffee and picks up the phone.

"Can I talk with Debbie please?" Scott requests the receptionist at his doctor's office. It's probably time that I ask about this drop in energy. He knows he's getting older, but maybe there's something the doctor can do to help out. "Hey Scott, who are you calling about this time?" Debby's voice is kind and playful. "Umm, me. I haven't been feeling well. Do you have anything open in your schedule?"

"Of course" the tone in Debby's voice changes to concern. Scott almost never comes in, and when he does it's serious. His cancer was in remission years ago, but with the history she doesn't want to take any chances. "How's tomorrow at three?"

"You're a saint, I'll take it." Scott says. "See you then."

He hangs up the phone. A moment later Sara returns. "Nurse Peggy said she'd take care of them. She took the bicillin out of the refrigerator to warm it up."

"Did you let her know that we already got blood from them?"

"Yes, and I gave it to her to send out. She said she'd do your paperwork, but you owe her a drink."

Scott chuckles "Deal, I hate doing the paperwork. Are they checked in?"

Sara looks down the hall "Not yet, I can still see them in the lobby."

"I hope they don't take off; patients have been known to do that." Scott leans back in his chair.

"Really, why would they come all the way over here and leave before getting treated?"

"Well, often the bad decisions that people make that get them infected with something affect other areas of their lives. So if they make poor decisions in one area they are likely to make poor decisions in other areas. These are generalizations of course, but a person who doesn't select partners wisely may also not select their careers wisely. If they don't take care of their bodies, they may not take care of their finances. And the same decisions that get people infected with disease can also cause unplanned pregnancies and substance abuse. It's all interconnected."

The description is over simplified, but apt. Sara appreciates the association and realizes that there are many contributing factors to disease spread. Poverty, education, culture, and many other characteristics affect how successfully disease is able to spread among people. The group of people they are working with now seem to be young, teens to twenties, high school education or lower, reside in one zip code, and are associated with crack use.

Looking at the generalization of the group, Sara can see why some people will be at higher risk than others in society.

Peggy passes Scott's office where the two investigators are talking. "I'm calling one back now. I'll tell you when I'm done." "Thank you Peggy, I appreciate you fitting them in." The nurse nods "It's what I'm here for." Peggy says half jokingly.

"Angela!" the call from the waiting area can be heard back to Scott's office. The young woman gets up from the hard plastic seats and meets the nurse in the hall. "Follow me back to room # 2." They walk back to the exam room where she will receive her injections.

Soon after entering the room, Angela emerges with an unhappy expression. Nurse Peggy walks her to Scott's office and uses a hand gesture to invite the woman into the investigator's room. Angela takes a seat next to Scott's desk and Sara closes the door to the office.

"What questions do you have?" Scott makes eye contact with the young lady. "Why did I have to get treated? Couldn't you just test me?" Scott nods, validating what the woman is saying. "You fit the description of someone who was exposed to Syphilis. I don't want to put off treatment until we get test results in case the test doesn't pick up the infection for some reason." Scott knows that with the recent exposure it's likely that her syphilis test would be negative, but he can't tell her about how recent the exposure is because it could violate James' confidentiality. Unlike police investigators,

Scott must walk a very tight line between informing patients about exposures and not disclosing any information that could lead them to identify someone who is infected.

"Who's the last person you had sex with?" Scott asks the young lady politely. He starts feeling tired again soon after asking the question. Maybe too much work.

"That fool in the lobby." She points in the direction of the waiting area. Scott goes on to ask follow up questions about her other partners. He focuses on the last few months knowing that he can identify social contacts even if they are not source spread candidates. The list is fairly extensive. Eight partners in the last 2 months. She doesn't know most of them. One of the men she tells Scott about matches the description of James, so Scott has greater confidence in the quality of information she's providing him with.

"How long have you been hook'n?" The question is a bit of a stretch, but Scott gets the sense, based on her description of the encounters with these men, that she is likely a prostitute. And the risk of offending her is worth the possibility of locating the Johns. One of them may have started this outbreak.

Startled by the question, but not offended, she responds "Just a few months." "So how many of these guys paid you for sex?" Scott follows up. "All of them. Except for Grimy. I just stay with him while I'm look'n for a place."

"Where do you meet these guys?" Scott needs locations so he has a starting place to find them. Prostitutes can be difficult to find, but Johns (men who pay prostitutes) can be almost impossible. "These one's came by Grimy's place." She points out the most recent four guys on Scott's pad. "These two I met up with at Cheever Park." Her candid responses are helpful but a little unsettling. Scott needs this information, but he also needs to talk with her about ways to prevent getting infected in the future. Her apathetic approach to casual sex may impair some of his ability to help her.

Angela answers the rest of Scott's questions with few problems. From the conversation the investigators understands that she's been using crack for about a year. She finances the habit through prostitution, and acquires her drugs from Grimy. It's all fairly straight forward. When asked about who Lawrence is having sex with she becomes more reluctant.

"We don't work with the police at all. Nothing you tell us is going to be used to prosecute anyone." Scott senses the need to distance himself from law enforcement officials. He makes it clear that the purpose of his investigations is to keep people from getting and spreading disease. It's a very different goal from that of police detectives.

"Grimy gives these hoes rock for pussy. They come and go. I don't really know them like that."

"Which of these women are your friends? How we can find them?"

"I said I don't know" Scott leaves the subject alone for now. He may revisit it later if Lawrence is less forthcoming.

"I want to thank you for talking with us, Angela. I know this wasn't an easy thing to do, but your help may save lives." The validation is welcomed. With no further questions she is excused to wait in the lobby until Scott and Sara are done talking with Lawrence.

Almost on cue, nurse Peggy calls on the office phone "He's ready for you." "Thanks Peggy, I'll be down shortly." Scott turns to Sara, "So what do you think?"

Sara shakes her head "I think we'll never figure out how these people got infected. There are so many partners and in a lot of cases almost nothing to go on. Look at this one." Sara points to the description of one of Angela's partners on Scott's pad. "How are we going to find unknown first name unknown last name with black hair, about medium height, drives either a Chevy or a Ford station wagon and met in the park?" Scott chuckles, "We call him Unk Unk for starters. Next we go to the park and look for this car and a guy who looks like this driving." Sara again looks at Scott intently, trying to determine if he is joking. He doesn't appear to be. "Let's see what Lawrence wants to tell us shall we?"

"I'll get him" Sara offers. She wants to stretch her legs from that last interview. The short walk down the hall helps a little. "Lawrence? We are ready for you." The exam room reeks of marijuana, cigarettes, and dirty feet. Sara's glad that the interview is taking place in Scott's office instead of hers. Lawrence follows Sara to Scott's office and he walks in and plops down in the open chair. Again the door is closed.

"You been look'n fo me hu."

"Several times, Lawrence" Scott acknowledges. "Did they swab you today?"

"Ya, nurse said I needed to get checked, you know, just to make sure."

"It's a good choice. Well, Sara's going to talk with you about partners and I'm going to be here in case I have additional questions."

Sara didn't expect to be thrust into the middle of an important part of this investigation at all, let alone without prior notice. She feels a little light headed and isn't sure if it is from the pressure of performing well or from the rancid stench.

"Lawrence, do you have any questions before we begin?"

Lawrence smiles displaying his yellow teeth and leans forward towards Sara "Call me Grimy, baby" he says with pride in his best smooth talking voice. Sara holds back her disgust from the revolting proposition well.

"Ok, Grimy, any questions about Syphilis?"

"Naw, I'm good."

"Who's the last person you've had sex with?"

"That bitch Angie out there."

"Ok, who else have you had sex with in the last year?

"Shit, I duno."

"Just try to remember the last couple of them, who were they?"

"Let's see, there's that bitch Tia…"

Sara interrupts him, having heard the term one too many times today. "Just for me, can you not call these ladies that? They are someone's sister, mother, and daughter. You wouldn't want someone to talk about a woman you cared about like that, right?" Leading questions are usually discouraged, but in this case the phrasing works well. That's probably because Lawrence is testing the young woman to see how far he can push her.

"Alright, so Tia, Becky, and, that's all the ones I have names for… Oh wait. That bitc…I mean punk Red's girl. What's her name? Chris I think. We hooked up few weeks back while Red was in Jail for DUI. You don't tell nobody bout this right?"

"Everything you tell me stays between us." Sara reassures the man.

"The rest of em, I couldn't tell you noth'n bout em. Just chicken heads I met up with on the street."

Sara conducts the rest of the interview well asking about his drug use, which he mostly denies other than weed, and his friends, which he either can't name, doesn't remember, or doesn't have depending on which version of the answer the investigator wants to pay attention to. Sara turns to Scott who had been listening intently to the discussion and asks "Did I miss anything?" To which Scott replies, "Always, but you did a good job. I don't have any questions. We'll need to talk with you again. You'll hear from either Sara or me when we get your results. Do you have any questions?"

Lawrence rubs his hands together quickly and asks "Can you drop me by the store? I need to pick up some things." Scott agrees, "I'll drop you and Angela off at the store, but I can't wait for you. You'll have to find a way home." The arrangement is acceptable to Lawrence and they leave the office. Angela is waiting for them in the lobby anxious to leave. "What took you so long?" She inquires of Lawrence. He doesn't reply, perhaps not wanting to discuss his business in the waiting area of the public health clinic. The four of them leave the clinic and get into Scott's car. Scott drives them to the closest grocery store, as agreed and drops the couple off at the front door. "Take care of yourselves. Talk with you later on." Scott says as they exit the car and make their way into the building.

He rolls down all of the car windows and the vehicle is filled with frigid, but fresh air. The smell drifts out of the car with a stubborn will. "I hope they don't decide to rob the place. I'd hate to be under suspicion for aiding an armed robbery." Scott says jokingly to Sara, who this time knows it's a joke. She hopes. Scott rolls the windows back up and he turns on the heat. The car still smells faintly of their latest passengers, but a couple of tree car fresheners and a little time should correct that. He makes his way towards Cheever Park.

"Where are we going?" inquires Sara. "Cheever to find your John" is the response.

Sara assesses "This should be interesting."

Scott's hopes are very low for finding this person, but since they are already in the field and close to the park it's worth a shot. If he makes enough trips there at the right times he may find the man in the station wagon.

Cheever Park is an unfortunate public works project. It was constructed to provide neighborhood kids a place to play, get some exercise, and be safe. But, it's deteriorated into a haven for drug dealers, prostitutes, thieves, and scoundrels of different varieties. There are very few children, even at this time of day, and the few that are here are either closely supervised by adults who appear to be overly aware of their surroundings or unsupervised miniature versions of the disreputable adults that frequent this place. Scott drives around the park slowly first looking for the car that fits the description Angela gave him. He spots a couple of possibilities, but no matching black haired man near the vehicles. Scott parks near the basketball courts and turns off the car's engine. "What are we doing?" Sara asks. "We are going to watch this car for a minute." Scott points out the car that most fits. "You'd be surprised at how much you can get by waiting." Scott adds to his response.

Scott and Sara sit in the car, protected from the cold by the intermittent heat that Scott permits from the Chevy. They watch prostitutes and Johns meet up and leave. Then see the prostitutes come back moments later only to get into another car and leave again. "I could make my whole career here" Scott points out. Sara realizes through this observation that that they will never run out of patients.

In addition to the prostitutes applying their trade, drug dealers are loitering around occasionally active when approached by a customer. The speed at which they conduct their business transaction is impressive. If someone isn't looking right at them, they would miss the whole deal. "This is a whole different world. It has different rules, different goals, different standards for success and failure. It's important to understand it so you know how to relate with your patients" Scott says The field trip is eye opening for Sara which alone makes it worth the time. But the investigators get a break as a man who fits the description of the one Angela gave them approaches the car they've been watching, in the company of one of the women they've been watching.

"There he is." Sara can hear the excitement in Scott's voice as he points out the man. Scott quickly gets out of the car and walks over to the guy. Scott is cautious not to approach him too close before announcing himself. "Excuse me." Scott calls to the man who looks back at Scott with a mix of fear and suspicion. The woman who had been accompanying the man turns around and walks away. "My name's Scott and I have important health information for you." Scott shows the man his identification badge. Not knowing if he believes the assertion, the man replies "What do you want?" as Sara joins Scott. Scott slowly approaches him while talking. "You may have been exposed to a very dangerous disease. I'd like to get you tested."

"What kind of disease?" The man seems shocked. Scott comes close enough to discuss the situation with some discretion. "Syphilis." Scott tells the new contact. "What?! How do you know this?"

Scott concedes that it's a fair question. "I can't tell you who told us because of confidentiality, but it's very important that we get you tested. If you have it we can treat you, if not than great. You'll know you don't have it."

"What do I have to do?" The man asks.

"Can you follow us to the health department? I'm driving the white Chevy over there" Scott points to his car. The man looks at the car, then Sara, who waves at him "Hi, I'm Sara, we work together."

"Ya, I'll follow you over there. When will I know something?"

"It'll take about a week. I'll call you as soon as I know your results though. What's your name?" Scott is compelled to ask for this information before leaving in case they are separated or the guy changes his mind en route. "Mike Simmons."

"Nice to meet you Mike. I'll get you in and out of the clinic as fast as possible."

Scott and Sara return to Scott's car. The Ford station wagon follows them closely the whole way to the clinic and both cars park in the lot.

Scott is pleased that Mike didn't get "lost" on the way. It's a good idea to test Mike for as many STDs as possible, but addressing his choices that subject him to disease is foremost on Scott's mind. Scott greets Mike at his car and the three of them travel up the sidewalk to the clinic entrance. Mike is wired. He appears panicked. His wide eyes scan the waiting area searching for people he knows, people who know him. Scott escorts Mike to the front desk where James greets him. "Good afternoon." James smiles, making eye contact with both men as they approach. Sara follows closely behind. "Hey James, Can you check him in?" Scott gestures to the apprehensive man who's still visibly uncomfortable. "Sure thing Scott. How's it hanging Sara?" James looks past Mike to greet the new staff member. The acknowledgment makes Sara feel more like part of the clinic's care team and she reciprocates. "I'm well James. Did you miss me?" "Of course" James responds to the playful riposte.

James changes his focus to Mike. "Good afternoon, sir. Do you have your ID with you?" Mike removes his wallet from his back pocket and produces a drivers license which he hands to James. "Thank you much. This won't take too long. Just need to check you in. Have you ever been seen here before."

"No" Mike says as if he's been accused of something.

"Ok, it'll just talk a little while to build you a chart. If you had been seen here before the check in process would be a little shorter is all. Can you fill out these forms please?" James hands Mike a clipboard with a few sheets of paper on them. "You can have a seat if you like while you're completing that. Just bring it back up when you're done." James hands Mike back his driver's license and continues to enter information into the clinic's system. Mike takes the clipboard and locates an acceptable seat in the waiting area. A pen is attached to the clipboard by a string and some tape. He begins filling out the forms.

Scott and Sara leave the reception desk and walk down the hall. Sara tells Scott "I need to get something from my office." He nods and she excuses herself continuing down the hall. Scott walks down the hall to the center of the main level to find Marge in the lab looking into a microscope. "Hey Marge, how's it going?"

"I'm blessed Scott, how are you doing?"

"I'm fine, just found some more work for you. He's checking in now." Scott motions to the reception desk.

"Thanks," sarcastically, "What's he need?"

"Well, a better class of friends I would guess. But I'd settle for testing. Can you give him the works?"

Smiling but not looking up from the microscope yet Marge replies, "Can do."

Marge looks up from the slide at Scott and he inquires, "What are you looking at?"

Marge steps away from the microscope and offers it to Scott, "You're the lab guy, you tell me."

Scott removes his glasses and presses his eyes into the microscope eye pieces. Egg shaped cells with small hairs flailing around swim around the slide. The organisms seem to almost understand that their lives are near the end. "Looks like trich. You got a good sample."

"Thanks, I aim to please." The nurse takes some pride in her work.

"Do you want me to talk to her?" Trichomoniasis isn't an infection that Scott usually does much with. The infection is very common and easily treatable. But women who have it may be at risk for other infections.

"No, you seem busy. I'll educate her and tell her to bring her partner in. If I need you to hunt some people down I know where to find you."

"You've got my number." Scott takes another look at the dying protozoa on the slide. Seeing them is interesting, but he doesn't miss working in the lab.

Meanwhile, Sara is at her office checking her e-mails. Mostly nothing of great interest, but one comes from her alma mater. She opens it and it's an invite from Dr. Rhodes who was a professor during her MPH program. He writes:

Dear Sara,

I hope this message finds you well. I'm sure you are a tremendous asset at the county health department. You were certainly among my better students and I regret that you were unable to attend the medical school program this semester. Your wit and knowledge would have greatly contributed to the students and staff here.

I hope you will consider reapplying for next year. The experience you gain at the public health clinic will strengthen your application, greatly improving your chances for acceptance into this program.

As always, keep in touch and contact me if you need anything,

Sincerely,

D. Rhoads, MD, MPH.

Sara closes the e-mail message and takes a moment to work through her feelings. She is still upset about not being accepted by the medical school. All she ever wanted to be was a doctor. The disappointment of receiving the rejection letter is refreshed by reading the message from her professor. Many of her friends were accepted. Sara was there when her roommate received her letter. It came before Sara's and as such was a harbinger of failure. She was happy for her friend. They had spent many nights studying together after school, drinking wine, and talking about their latest romantic interests. Sara produces as sarcastic smile. Maybe if there was less wine and talking and more study she could have gotten the chance to be a doctor. Sara's other class mates went on to internships at the CDC, doctoral programs, the military, US Public Health Service, FEMA, and a whole host of other stellar career tracks. She came here. Many applications were submitted, but the local health department was the only call she got. Sara remembers hesitating to even apply for the low paying, dead end position at the clinic. At the time she put in the application she thought of it as the tail end of public health. That perception has changed over the last couple of days. Scott told her when she came to work here that "This is where public health is done. Not at the CDC, not at FEMA, and not in academia or even at the state. The local health departments around the country do the bulk of preventing disease, maintaining health, educating the public. The other places create rules and collect data. They provide money and support us. But we do the work." Sara is beginning to see that and realizes for the first time since she arrived that she's a part of something special and important.

Sara contemplates reapplying to the medical school, or perhaps another one. But she knows she doesn't have to make a decision right now. In fact, right now there is Syphilis to stop and she's late to get to Scott's office.

Scott is looking over some notes as Sara reaches the office. He looks up from the pad at Sara "Is everything ok?" he asks sensing that his coworker is troubled.

"Ya" She tells Scott with conviction still redirecting her focus from the past to the present.

"Mike isn't out of the exam room yet. Shouldn't be long though. We are going to focus pretty heavily on a risk assessment and a reduction strategy with him." Scott informs Sara of the plan which involves learning what Mike is doing that could get him infected, and coming up with ways to avoid getting infected in the future.

"You mean like not picking up crack prostitutes in the park?" Sara says sarcastically. Scott laughs. "Something like that."

Mike is brought to Scott's office by nurse Marge after about fifteen minutes. He still appears anxious and expresses concern for being infected.

Scott begins the interview by asking him, "How are you doing?"

"I just want to know if I got something." Mike rubs his knees and fidgets.

"We'll know more after we get your test results back. I want to talk with you some about what's going on and see if we can't help you. What do you think you did to put yourself at risk for getting Syphilis?" Scott's words may seem condescending, but the tone and body language is refined to express true concern for the patient's well being.

"Hooking up with these girls that I met in the park I guess." Mike admits. Sara looks at Scott to receive validation but receives none.

"How many girls have you picked up in the last year Mike?"

"Maybe five?" Mike lies to the investigator. Probability indicates that finding this guy by chance in the park on one of the few occasions he claims to go is very low. Scott believes he may be there almost every day.

"Who are some of the main ones that you pick up?"

"Just whoever is there that I like. Sometimes it's the same girl, I think."

Probing for additional information, Scott follows up the question. "OK, what do they look like, what part of the park are they located in..." Collecting descriptive and locating information continues for what seems like an eternity to the weary man.

"How often do you use condoms with these girls you pick up?"

"I don't use condoms. Can't find any that fit." Mike forces himself to laugh at the joke, but his anecdote is not received with the anticipated response by the investigators. Scott writes on his pad "Condoms too small" so that he can come back to the subject.

"What about your main girl, who is she?"

"I don't have one. I'm single." Mike asserts. Scott writes this information down on the pad also.

"How would you feel if you were told you had a STD?" The question has been on Mike's mind ever since meeting Scott and Sara in the park.

"I'd feel bad, dirty. I'd hope it's one I can get rid of."

"How would being infected with something you can't get rid of affect your life?" Scott follows up his previous question to prime the patient for the upcoming plan to reduce his risk.

"It would be bad. I'd have to change a lot of things. It would be bad…" The man looks down and shakes his head. He's contemplating something. Scott suspects that he's probably in a relationship, maybe even married, but that isn't the focus right now.

"What do you think you can do to keep yourself from getting infected?" Scott and Sara both have obvious ideas they can give Mike. But in order for him to truly change what he's doing he needs to have ownership of the idea. It has to come from him.

"I could ask the girls if they have something" he offers. Sara's frustration level increases while Scott expected a response similar to this.

"Talking with your partners is a good idea. What else?"

"I should get tested more often."

Scott nods, affirming the idea of routine testing for this man. "Getting tested is also a good idea. That way if you did get infected you can know about it before it becomes a major health problem. But testing doesn't keep you from getting infected. Now you've mentioned that you have problems finding condoms that fit. Have you tried the large or extra large sizes? We have some here I can give you."

"I didn't know they made different sizes. I guess I can try those out."

"Why do you go to the park to meet girls?"

"A friend of mine told me about it. It's just easier and faster than try'n to meet girls the usual ways."

"I'm not giving you relationship advice, but have you tried dating in the past?"

"Ya, sometimes I just want something quick. The girls at Cheever are cheap and they are always there."

"They may have STDs though, Mike. If they are having sex with you without condoms they may be having sex with other people without protection."

Mike's face sours. "Ewww." Envisioning all of the men who've had sex with the prostitutes makes Mike feel a little queasy. They made him feel special, but he wasn't. Sara thinks to herself that this is so obvious, but she remembers Scott telling her that this is a different world. She listens intently; the real life drama of the STD clinic is better than television.

"So what are some of the other things you can do to keep from getting infected?"

"I know you want me to say that I won't go to the park. But I can't tell you that I won't. Well…I can tell you that, but I'd be lying."

Scott responds to the statement "I just want to make sure that you have all the information you need to make an informed decision."

Scott goes on to educate him about diseases he can get by having sex with the prostitutes at Cheever Park. The list is extensive and Mike seems a little overwhelmed by the sheer quantity of STDs in the community. Scott talks with Mike about partners and the need to get them tested. Of course Mike doesn't know anyone he's had sex with lately leaving Scott with no one he can contact. Mike's best advice to Scott is to test everyone in the park.

The idea has merit. He jots that suggestion down on his pad "Outreach testing at Cheever Park."

Scott goes over the risk reduction plan one more time with Mike before he leaves. "Ok, so you've decided to ask the women you meet in the park if they have a STD, and to try to use condoms when you have sex with them?"

"Ya, I'll try it out."

"What problems do you see with doing this plan."

Mike laughs "Asking them if they got something might be weird, but I guess I'll know if they do how they answer." Scott agrees. "That's true, if they know. A lot of times they may not have symptoms."

"Well, I'm going to definitely try using the condoms."

"Sounds good. Do you have any questions?" Scott concludes.

"No I'm good. Thank you."

"No problem. Call me if you have any questions and here is a variety pack of condoms with different sizes." Scott hands Mike a small paper sack full of condoms.

"Ok" Mike takes the bag of condoms and puts them in his jacket pocket. "Thanks again." He leaves the office and exits the clinic feeling empowered by the testing and the conversation with Scott.

"What a mess!" Sara exclaims to Scott. "What kind of a risk reduction plan is that?" Scott understands her frustration. "It's a different world. We don't know what all is going on with him. Maybe some mental illness, likely substance abuse, sex addiction. What would you have him do, join a convent?"

"Not have sex with hookers in the park!" Sara responds.

"Everyone who has sex is at some risk for STDs. Everyone. I've seen people who find out that they are not in a monogamous relationship because they get infected with something. No one is exempt. So what level of risk people put themselves at is a matter of personal choice. I want to help them reduce the risk as much as they can tolerate, but in the end, they have to live their lives and they won't do it according to what you or I think is acceptable or not." Sara listens, still amazed at what some people find acceptable.

"There is no norm. What you and I think is acceptable, someone else thinks is bad, dangerous, risky, or sinful. Who's right? Who's wrong? It's up to people to decide for themselves. And that guy" Scott points towards the lobby, "has a plan to go from having sex with prostitutes without condoms to talking with them first and using protection. And he got tested. That's huge!" Sara realizes that there is a lot to learn about this job. She wonders if she'll stick around long enough to learn it.

"So what's next?" Sara changes the subject.

"Well, we have about three days' worth of work to do and about three hours to do it in." Scott examines his list of contact to the Syphilis case. "Let's head back to the field. We'll see if we can find Pritchard and Dustin." Sara strains her memory to recall who those people are. Scott notices the perplexed look on Sara's face. "They are Rose's partners." Scott reminds her. "I wouldn't remember either if it weren't for my notes." Sara feels a sense of relief and decides to start taking her own notes so she can keep up.

The two gather their belongings once again and leave the clinic to find the exposed men.

Scott drives the two of them to the first location, Dustin's half way house. Scott's been there before. Crime and STDs are common bedfellows. The house is a single floor multi room dwelling with sparse landscaping. The covered porch has several wooden chairs and benches. Two of the seats are occupied by residents who are smoking outside of the house. The gentleman are older, perhaps in their sixties. The one on the bench is wearing a jean jacket with denim pants and a ball cap with a Los Angeles Lakers emblem. He has a scraggly grey white beard and thick rimmed brown glasses. The other is sitting on a chair leaning back with his hands on the back of his head and legs spread apart. He appears to be very comfortable. He is wearing a red windbreaker with khaki pants and black boots. Sara and Scott approach the house with their pads and clip boards appearing very much like sales representatives.

One of the residents, who is seated on a wooden bench, calls to them as they approach the property. "We don't want none!" Scott smiles and says to himself "That's more true than you know."

"We are looking for Mr. Dustin Evens." Scott leaves it at that. Asking if they know who he is, if he's there, or if he's available gives the men an easy out. If they say no, than he's cut off. This way they have to provide a response. Many people will hesitate to lie to him, and if they attempt he can usually get an idea of what the truth may be.

"He aint here." The other responds.

"When will he be back?" Scott asks the man.

They look at each other and laugh at what appears to be an inside joke. "He ain't com'n back." The comment is followed by more laughter.

"Where did he go?" Sara follows up Scott's question.

"Five O picked him up last night. Umm Hmm, drug him out of here in irons."

"Do you know where they took him?" Sara again follows up.

"I'm guess'n the county. Don't know what he done. Might not be there long."

"Thank you" Scott says to the men. Sara and Scott return to the car. "Feel like going to jail?"

Scott calls his contact at the county jail from his cell phone. "Hi Eric this is Scott."

"Scott, what's up man? What have you been up to?"

"Same old, you know…stamping out disease. Hey, I'm on my way over. Need to talk with Dustin Evens. Police should have brought him in last night." Scott doesn't discuss patient information over his cell for security reasons, and Eric doesn't ask for specifics. If Scott is coming over now it's serious and Eric will do everything he can to help."

"Got you my man, I'll tell the guards to expect you."

Sara's never been to jail before. From what she's seen on TV it's a scary looking place filled with unhappy guards and prisoners. That's only part of the truth, as she will soon see.

The two arrive at the county jail and park in the visitors parking. "You'll need to leave your cell phone, purse, and keys in the car." Scott advises Sara. She take her phone out of her purse and places it in the console. Scott looks down at it. "We'll need to lock this stuff up." He opens the glove compartment. Scott removes his cell phone and pocket knife and places them into the glove box. "The prisoners who are on minimum security may come out to the parking lot to clean up. You don't want them to see anything in the car that they'll want. You should put your purse in the trunk." Sara does as Scott suggests, though she feels naked without her purse and cell phone. "Bring your ID." Scott advises her and she retrieves it before Scott closes the trunk.

The investigators approach the jail. The facility is a large brown brick building surrounded by a high chain link fence topped with constantino wire coiled in large loops. The main entrance leads into a large waiting area with soft benches and a television that's playing cartoons. The pair walk up to the duty desk and greet the guard who is sitting behind thick glass. "I'm Scott, this is Sara. We are with the health department. Eric said he'd let you know we were coming."

The officer on duty passes Scott a log book through a small opening at the base of the window. "Sign in there. Do you have your IDs?" Scott and

Sara both hand the guard their badges and he places them in a rack against the wall. The guard slides two clip- on numbered badges through the opening and asks the visitors to write the badge numbers next to their name on the logbook.

After signing in Scott removes his shoes and his belt. The door next to the guard opens and he hands each of them a basket. Scott looks at Sara, "It's like the airport." Enough said. Sara removes her ear rings, necklace, watch, and shoes. She places them in the plastic container and puts the container on the x-ray conveyer belt. The guard views the items as they pass though then allows the health department workers to pass through the metal detector. Scott enters first passing without incident. Sara follows after.

Beeep! The machine pings.

Sara walks back through. She looks herself over inventorying her attire unable to find the offending article. The guard offers his assistance. "This thing is pretty sensitive; it's probably just your underwire. Come over here and I'll wand you." The wanding is a bit more intrusive than she feels is necessary, but it confirms the guard's suspicions. "Wait over there." He directs them to a bench against the wall near the entrance to the first hall. "Eric will be down to get you soon."

The walls of the jail appear to be cinder block painted white. The heavy steel doors are battleship gray and the clanging of their movement echoes throughout the facility. The place appears unusually quiet. The guard is playing a radio at a low volume, and the sporadic chatter over the hand held radios provides breaks in the silence. "I'd like for you to talk to him." Scott tells Sara. She's pleased to receive sufficient warning this time and begins to organize what she wants to say.

Light footsteps are heard walking down the hall towards the guard station. The guard buzzes the door open and Eric enters the area. Eric is a tall man with sharp features and a lean build. He is wearing blue scrubs with tennis shoes. "Hi Scott, who's this?"

"Eric, Sara…Sara, Eric. He's the guy to come to when you need something at the jail."

"Which is all the time" Eric interjects his opinion. "Not my fault your prisoners become my patients." Scott retorts jokingly.

"Follow me, I'll give you the nickel tour." Eric motions for the investigators to come with him and they comply. They walk through the first of many security doors which close with a loud clank behind them. The weight of the heavy locks are made evident by the imposing sound.

"The clinic is this way." Eric leads them through three more security doors; each increases the distance of the investigators from freedom. It takes a few minutes to reach the clinic even though it's a short distance from the security desk. The progress is hampered because the trio is forced to wait at each security door to be unlocked remotely by a guard. As they approach the clinic a prisoner is heard screaming in his cell. The words are unintelligible, and he appears to be alone. None of the other prisoners or guards in the area seem concerned by the outbursts. Prisoners are accompanied by large uniformed men and stick together in tight groups. A few of them glance over at the visitors with angry expressions, but none say anything to them as they pass by. The guards greet Eric who passes among them easily. "Here we are."

The group reaches the infirmary which is larger than Sara had imagined. It has a reception area similar to the health department's. A woman in her mid twenties sits at the desk which is cluttered with patient charts. "Looks like you've been busy." Scott observes.

Eric agrees, "Sometimes I think prisoners are the sickest people in the world. Guess they need to take full advantage of this free health care while they can. And take advantage they do." Eric asks the guard next to the check in desk to have Scott's patient brought to the clinic. The heavy set man, whose uniform is stressed to its limits agrees to Eric's request. He calls over the radio "Smith, they are ready for Dustin." The response is received quickly. "Roger that, en route."

Eric shows Sara and Scott to the exam room they will be using. "What do you need from me?"

"Can you get a Syphilis and HIV test on him?" Scott requests. He would have drawn the blood himself, but getting his test kit past security is more trouble than it's worth.

"Sure thing."

"We may need to treat him. It'll depend on what info I get from him during the interview." Scott advises Eric.

"OK, just let me know. He should be here soon."

Eric leaves and Scott and Sara wait in the exam room for the guards to bring Dustin in. The wait is long. For reasons unknown to the two of them Dustin doesn't arrive at the exam room for at least a half an hour. "Here he is." The guard presents the patient to the investigators. The sudden arrival after a long period of boredom jolts the public health workers into action.

"Hi Dustin, come on in." Scott invites the man to a chair.

"Do you need me to stay?" the burly man asks Scott.

"No, we'll be fine." The guard leaves and Scott closes the door to the exam room.

Scott gestures to Sara and she introduces the pair. "My name is Sara, this is Scott. We are with the health department."

"What's going on?" Dustin inquires.

"We are conducting a public health investigation and came here to tell you that you may have been exposed to Syphilis." The patient retains a flat affect. "So what?" Dustin sits back in his seat apparently unconcerned about the news of his possible affliction. "It's curable right?"

"Syphilis is. But it is also a very dangerous infectious disease. If it goes untreated than it can lead to some very serious health problems."

"So treat me." The patient's simplistic understanding of what Sara is trying to communicate frustrates the young investigator.

"We'll get you tested today, but I need to talk with you some more so I can better evaluate how we need to proceed with your medical care." Sara removes the picture cards from the back of her tablet. "After getting infected with Syphilis it takes about three weeks to develop a painless sore." She shows Dustin a picture of a few primary lesions. "Have you seen anything like this on yourself or any of your partners?"

"No, that's nasty. It's on the tongue in this picture. You can get Syphilis in your mouth?" Dustin acts disgusted by the card.

"The sore appears where ever the bacteria enter the body. Usually where you come in contact with someone else's sore." Sara educates the patient.

"Well I ain't been lick'n nobodies Syphilis sore!"

Sara continues "The sore lasts for about three weeks and then goes away. At that point the bacteria is starting to travel throughout the body and a few weeks later a person can get a rash," Sara shows Dustin a picture of a rash on a person's body. "The rash can also be on the palms of the hands and soles of the feet. These are called palmer planter rashes. Have you seen anything like this on yourself or any of your partners?"

"Nope, but that's what Grimy's got." Dustin points to the picture of the rash on a person's hands. Can I get Syphilis by touch'n that rash?" Now he acts concerned.

"No, the rash isn't contagious. Have you seen a rash like this on anyone else?"

"No, just him. I told him that shit wasn't right and he needed to get checked. Dumb ass."

Sara writes the notes on her pad regarding Dustin's association with Lawrence so that she can come back to it.

"Later, as the bacteria spread it damages the tissues where it ends up. Sometimes that tissue is in the lungs, the heart or the brain. This is how Syphilis causes a lot of damage to someone who has it. It can be life threatening."

"Dang," Dustin seems to grasp the severity of the situation. "You're saying I might have this?"

"Yes, it's possible."

"Who told you about me?"

"I can't tell you that because it involves someone else's medical information. Just like I can't give someone your information, I can't give you someone else's."

"But I need to know so I don't mess with them again."

"I understand that it's frustrating to not know who may have exposed you, but what's most important right now is to make sure you're ok and that the infection doesn't spread."

"I need to know who this is. You've got to tell me. It's my right to know who gave up my name."

"Well, I can tell you that it's someone who cares enough about you to let us get you taken care of. Beyond that I can't give you any information."

Dustin thinks about that for a moment and either accepts it or concedes that he won't convince the young investigator to give him the information.

"We also need to talk about the people you've had sex with. We need to get them tested." Sara continues.

"Shit, if you aint tell'n me who named me, I aint tell'n you bout nobody else." Dustin attempts to barter with information.

"We know you may have been exposed to Syphilis, but if you're at risk for Syphilis than you may be at risk for other sexually transmitted diseases. Locating and testing your partners may be the only way we find out you've been exposed to something else."

"I aint tell'n you shit." The defiant inmate declares.

"Syphilis can kill people if it goes untreated. And pregnant women can develop serious birth defects. I'm sure you don't want to have dead or deformed children on your conscience. Especially since one of these kids could be yours." Sara attempts to make eye contact with him and makes a compelling case for him to tell her who else may be affected, but to no avail.

"Fuck em. They'll figure it out."

The rest of the interview progresses smoothly. Sara educates him about the tests, treatment, and talks with him some more about symptoms. She tries a few more times to get him to name partners but is unsuccessful. She concludes the interview and calls for the guard. Eric follows the guard back to the exam room. "So are we treating him?" Sara looks at Scott. Scott looks at the prisoner, "No, we'll wait. If he's positive he'll figure it out." He and Sara leave the exam room and Eric walks in with his blood kit.

"So why aren't we treating him?" Sara asks Scott. "The guy is a first class A hole, but we can't just let him walk around with Syphilis." Scott responds "The exposure was long ago enough where all we have to do is test him. He doesn't have any symptoms. Treating him with antibiotics is unnecessarily. He could have an allergic reaction which could endanger his life. Besides, he is incarcerated. This is a very controlled environment. People do manage to have sex in prison, but not usually in the county. He'll be ok and we know where to find him if he does come back positive."

"So what did I do wrong?" Sara asks as the guard escorts them down the hall to the security desk.

"You mean besides not getting any partners?"

Feeling a little like salt was rubbed in her would. "Ya."

"Nothing, you did a good job."

"Ok, so why wouldn't he tell me?"

"We use our motivators to get people to talk. You did a great job with that. But in the end it's up to them whether of not to tell you anything. The reasons for that are numerous and range from the simple to the very complex. With him, we know he's a criminal so he may have some anti-social disorder. He seemed to get into a power struggle with you. When he couldn't intimidate, badger, barter, or coerce you into giving him what he wanted, he decided not to give you want you wanted."

"So he's just being childish."

"Maybe. It's possible that he's hiding something too. Maybe he's having sex with men, children, one of his friend's girlfriends. There's something he doesn't want us to know."

"What now?"

"We go find the next one. Hopefully." Scott and Sara reach the security station and pass back through the metal detector. It goes off again for both of them which is a minor annoyance and irrelevant. The guard hands them the log book so they can sign out. "Badges please." Scott and Sara remove the visitor badges attached to their shirts. "I'm glad you reminded me," Scott tells the guard. "I've got three of these at home." The guard fails to find the humor in the joke, which is literally true. Scott has at least three of these things. "Here you go." The humorless jail guard returns Scott and Sara's IDs to them and takes back the log book. The two depart the jail and get back in Scott's Chevy.

The day has mostly escaped, but Scott chooses to try one last field visit before going home. Pritchard lives about ten minutes from here, or he did 6 years ago when he received his last immunization from the health department. Scott enters the address into his smart phone's GPS and follows the directions to the destination, the female computerized voice guiding him the whole way. He's amazed at how often the computer doesn't know its left from its right. The designers of this system still have a lot of work to do.

They reach the house, a yellow single level with white trim. There's a large tree in the center of the well maintained yard. "Too well maintained for a crack addict" Scott thinks to himself. Hopefully the parents are still here and at least know where to find Pritchard. The two investigators walk down the narrow walk way to the front door. The curtains are open and the house gives off a warm comfortable vibe. Sara knocks on the door.

After a moment a woman comes to the door. She is maybe late forties, early fifties. She addresses the visitors "How can I help you?" Scott looks at Sara and Sara turns to answer the woman. "Hi ma'am, we are looking for Pritchard Wallace." The woman sighs, "Is he in some sort of trouble again?" Sara assures the woman, "No ma'am, we just need to talk with him about a very important health matter."

"Health matter? What's going on?" The woman expresses a great deal of concern.

"I really can't tell you because of confidentiality, but it's very important that I speak with him."

"But I'm his mother." The woman justifies her curiosity by asserting her relationship.

"I'm sorry ma'am, I really can't tell you. I'd get in trouble."

The woman sighs again and looks over the investigators. "Pritchard!" she calls inside the house for her son. "What mom?" A man in his twenties comes into view. He's tall and thin with clean clothes and well maintained hair. His appearance is not what Scott or Sara were expecting. Scott thinks to himself "Another lesson about assuming."

"These people are looking for you." The woman points to Sara and Scott. Scott waves and Sara introduces them. "Can we talk outside for a moment?" Sara asks Pritchard with a polite tone.

"Sure" Pritchard closes the door while his mother looks on from inside the house.

Sara keeps her voice low to avoid the eavesdropping parent. "Pritchard, your name came up in a Syphilis interview and we need to test you."

The man looked surprised "Me?"

"Yes. I know this isn't the news you wanted to hear. We can get some blood from you to see if you're infected and then treat you if necessary."

"I know who it is. It's Rose right?"

"I really can't tell you anything about who named you because of confidentiality."

"You don't have to tell me. I've only been with one person in a year."

Sara talks with him about the signs and symptoms of Syphilis and it's dangers. Pritchard is respectful and at least appears to be compliant, though Scott would remind her that all patients lie. Pritchard agrees to let the investigators test him and invites them inside. "What do they want you for?" Pritchard's mom inquires of him.

"They said I might have Syphilis" Pritchard candidly answers his mother. Sara is surprised by the answer, but it makes testing him easier. "Oh my Lord! Syphilis? Pritchard I told you to leave those hoochies alone. You need to wrap it up! Lord I swear if you get some girl pregnant... I'm not chang'n no diapers!" Scott believes Pritchard's mom has developed a good risk reduction strategy. Sara feels awkward witnessing this family interaction.

"Mom! Just hush. We don't need all that."

"Can we use this table?" Scott asks and points to a large table with wooden chairs around it in the dining room.

"Sure" Pritchard replies and leads the two guests into the large dining room. The house is well furnished with many shelves full of various knick knacks. There are also many plaques and mirrors on the walls many of which make reference to Scripture or have other religious verbiage. The furniture is predominantly wood, especially in the dining room. There is a pleasant sent of pine and lemon. Pritchard and the investigators take seats at the large table and Scott removes items from his blood kit to collect the specimen. "Which arm would you like?"

Prichard lays his left arm against the table in preparation of the blood draw. Scott takes only a few moments to collect the sample. The mother hovers outside the room refusing to vacate the area so that Pritchard can speak with the health department workers. Sara talks with Pritchard about the disease and how to prevent infection in the future. She asks about partners again, but he maintains that he's only had the one in the last year. They conclude the visit and excuse themselves.

"I'll give you a call at the number you left on the registration form when we get your test results back. Thank you much for meeting with us." Scott tells the man.

"Thank you for coming by." Pritchard reciprocates the sentiment.

"Thank you for letting us into your home Ma'am" Sara says to Pritchard's mother. The mother waves, still concerned about her son. The investigators leave the house and walk back to the car.

"Not a bad way to end our day" Scott says to Sara. They open the doors to the car and climb inside. "Now back to the clinic."

The two drive back to the clinic, about twenty minutes in rush hour. It's half past five and they find the facility closed, the staff has gone home. "We'll turn this stuff in in the morning" Scott tells Sara. "Here, hold onto the blood and bring it with you when you come back."

"Yuck! What am I supposed to do with that?" Sara points at the container holding the tube of potentially infected blood.

"Put it in your refrigerator" Scott advises her.

"Good night Scott." Sara turns away and walks back to her car. Her non verbal communication profoundly stating her objection to Scott's suggestion.

"Good night Sara." Scott calls after her. Scott watches her get into her car and pull away before he gets into his own car and pulls out of the clinic parking lot. He's tired. "Been a long day" Scott says to himself. On the trip home Scott unwinds listening to some jazz from his MP3 player. Big band helps clear the mind and relax the soul. When he reaches his apartment Scott takes all of the patient information and the sample out of his car and up to his apartment. He has some difficulty climbing the stairs but reaches the second floor after exerting himself. "It may be time to get a first floor apartment" he comments. Scott enters his apartment, sets his brief case on the table by the still dirty dishes from this morning's breakfast. He goes to the refrigerator and removes a beer from the six pack within, and sets the patients specimen next to his eggs.

As he does every evening, Scott dials his daughters' phone number before they go to bed. The phone rings a couple of time. "Hi daddy." the young lady's voice comes over the earpiece clearly, warming Scott's heart. "Hi baby, how are you?"

"I'm ok, I received my test grade today from history." Monica, Scott's youngest daughter pauses. "It's an A." He can hear the smile in her voice. The child had been struggling a little since the beginning of the year. She doesn't like her history teacher Mrs. Hildabranch, but it seems as though Monica has warmed up to her somewhat as the semester has gone on. Scott encourages his child "Good job baby! How have your studies been going in the other classes?"

"Umm, pretty good,…better than they were anyway." The child qualifies her academic success in an attempt to conceal the mostly average performance. Scott of course picks up on this. "What have you been doing to improve your grades?"

"Dad! You're not supposed to use your work questions on me. The open end ones." She giggles as she was caught trying to evade the investigator's line of questioning.

"She is so smart," Scott thinks to himself. "OK, well do better. I love you."

"Love you too daddy. Want to talk to Ellisa?"

"No, but I'd love to talk <u>with</u> her." Scott corrects Monica's grammar.

The child lets out a frustrated breath and cups the receiver. "Ellisa! It's Dad!"

"Hello?" Ellisa answers as if she doesn't know Scott is on the phone.

"Hi baby, how are you."

"I'm fine Dad, just in the middle of doing my homework." She states impatiently.

Scott shakes his head and puts his hand over his face thinking to himself "Teenagers!" He continues talking with his daughter, "So how's school going?"

"It's about the same as yesterday."

"Good," Scott doesn't know what else to say at this point and doesn't want to force a conversation with her. "Well, have a good night, I love you."

"Love you Dad, good night." The response is hurried and the phone goes dead.

Scott has a seat on the couch and puts his feet on the ottoman. He takes a few swallows of beer and turns on the TV. "What a really long day." His eyes become too heavy to keep open and he falls asleep.

Chapter 5

Sara walks into the clinic at 7:55 in the morning. She had a great night's sleep, probably caused by the busy day of chasing disease. She approaches the counter to find the administrative assistants already there. "Good morning Sandy, James." The pleasant tone of Sara's voice is in sharp contrast to her previously somber morning moods. She's excited to be at work today, curious about what new things she'll learn and people she'll meet. "Good morning Sara, how was your evening?" James asks seemingly genuinely interested.

"It was great. I went to bed at nine." She laughs. The statement made her sound like she was 50. James shrugs "If you say so. Early to bed early to rise and such." Sandy participates by offering insight into her evening "I was up till almost midnight."

James interjects jokingly "You don't have to give us any details."

"Not like that you perv. I was reading this new book about a South American cop who's trying to take down the cartel, but he falls in love with the gangster's daughter…"

"Ya," James says with a hint of sarcasm and eye rolling, "I can see why that would keep you up. I was with you till you brought up the love thing. Hasn't the Romeo and Juliet thing been done enough?"

"You don't mess with a classic." Sandy offers the advice.

Sara finds the conversation interesting albeit juvenile. She has a lot of work that needs to get done today and excuses herself. "Well you two have fun, we'll be in touch soon."

She briskly walks down the hall to find Scott's door still closed. She knocks, but there's no answer. She hears the distinctive sound of high heels striking tile floor approaching and looks towards the source of the noise to find Ann walking towards her. "Good morning Sara. Scott will be in late this morning."

"OK, we are working on a Syphilis outbreak, I'll wait till he gets here." Sara suggests.

"Can you finish your modules please? We need to have your basic training completed before sending you to the Passport to Partner Services course."

"I'll do that now."

"Thank you Sara, Scott should be here in an hour or so." Ann walks towards the reception desk, the sound of her heels fading into the hall. Sara walks back to her office and turns on her computer. It takes a couple minutes to boot up, but she's soon back to reading a seemingly endless stream of text from the online training module. Being a good student, she's able to quickly grasp the information presented in this basic training course, but her attention keeps changing from the computer to ideas about the investigation. She decides that maybe some coffee will help.

Scott breaches the clinic doors about an hour later. He's unaccustomed to coming in late, but overslept. "Morning Scott" Sandy greets her coworker as he comes in. Concern is heard in her voice. She's never known Scott to come in late before unless he was doing field visits before the work day started. "Morning," Scott replies "Is Ann here?"

"She's in her office. Told us you'd be a little late. Everything OK?" Sandy's concern evident in her tone.

"Ya, I'm fine" Scott shoots the receptionist a grin "Still saving lives." Scott leaves the desk and makes his way down the hall. He drops off his bag and jacket in his office then proceeds to the lab where he places the sample from yesterday afternoon's late blood draw into the clinic refrigerator. The courier will collect it in a couple of hours and deliver it to the state laboratory. Continuing his rounds, Scott walks down the hall and reaches Sara's office. "I'm going to meet with Ann, then we'll be off." Sara looks up from her computer. Scott's voice snapped her out of a study trance and it took her a second to process the interruption. "Sure thing" she replies, happy to get away from the computer training again.

Scott climbs the steps and makes his way down the hall on the second level towards Ann's office. He finds her door closed. That's atypical for her because she likes to keep it open unless she's on a call. He walks back down the hall to the employee lounge where he gets a small paper cup and fills it will coffee. The coffee doesn't seem as good today. It fails to hit the spot that it usually does. Scott examines the paper cup, maybe it's because it's not in his cup. Maybe it's because he already feels energized from a good night's sleep. Scott hears the door open from down the hall and follows the sound to Ann's office. "Good morning Ann" he greets his long time boss and friend. "Good morning Scott, how are you feeling?"

"I'm feeling good now. I've got a doctor's appointment this afternoon though. Just a check up."

Ann's known Scott long enough to know he doesn't go to the doctor unless he has to, but trusts his judgment when it comes to his health. He isn't one to complain about ailments and will let her know if there's something to worry about.

"Tell me about the investigation" Sara leans forward in her seat and listens intently. The patient interaction is what she misses most about leaving nursing and going into administration.

Scott takes a seat across from her desk. "It's going well. We are finding some cases, getting people tested. Sara and I are going back out this morning to locate a couple more contacts."

"How's she doing" Ann inquires of the new hire.

"Great, she's going to be a good investigator. I've had her talk with some patients already. She's picking up this stuff fast."

"Good to hear. Well, let me know if I can help. I'd love to get out of the office for a while." Ann offers, but she realizes Scott likely won't accept the help. Even if he does need it.

"I think we've got this right now. Thanks though." Scott stands and excuses himself. Ann watches him walk out of the office hoping he will be alright.

Scott swigs the coffee, more out of habit than enjoyment and walks downstairs.

As he passes Sara's office Scott again interrupts her studies "Meet me in my office and we'll go over the plan for today."

"Ok, just let me finish this section and I'll meet you there."

Scott nods and returns back to his office.

Sara works on developing her carpal tunnel syndrome as she clicks her way through the current section of the module. It takes her about five minutes to complete the test at the end, which she easily passes. She prints the results, e -mails a copy to Ann, and closes her computer. Grabbing her jacket and bag she leaves the office and goes to Scott's.

When she gets to Scott's office he is rummaging through some boxes stored inconspicuously. He produces a small cooler from one of the larger boxes on the floor. "Here is it" he exclaims "It's your new blood kit." He hands the dusty coleman to Sara.

She accepts it, wiping the dust from the top and sides of it "Thanks." Sara looks into the box of miscellaneous items Scott's collected over the years and pull out a particularly strange one. "Pink snake?" she asks Scott holding up a plush pink toy cylindrical in shape and coiled with eyes on its face. "It's a spirochete" Scott corrects her. She reexamines the stuffed toy. Having just completed the chapter on Syphilis she recognizes the item as resembling the shape of the bacteria that causes Syphilis. "The CDC came out with a whole line of stuffed animal pathogenic micro-organisms years ago. That's the Syphilis one." Sure enough, the tag on the creature read CDC, Syphilis. "Scott smiles "It's yours, take it."

"Thanks," Sara looks at the creature still contemplating the usefulness of such an item. "I'll cherish it always," she continues with just a slight hint of sarcasm.

"Let's go by the lab and fill up your new blood kit. Hey, we might even get lucky and find some patients to practice on." Scott and Sara take the empty cooler to the lab. Scott begins rifling through the lab supplies to stock the blood bag. Sara takes the dirty bag to the sink and washes it thoroughly. While pilfering the laboratory supplies Scott notices a clinic nurse pass by. "Hey Marge, if you get one that needs a blood draw can you come get us? Sara needs some practice."

"Of course Scott. Thank you for taking the supplies from the lab and not my exam room this time." The nurse uses this as an opportunity to express her displeasure with Scott's last restocking mission. "You're welcome" Scoot calls after the nurse who's departed down the hall.

Scott finds all of the supplies he needs, and Sara cleans and dries the blood kit. He gives the supplies to Sara who neatly organizes them and places them into her new blood kit.

As luck would have it a patient is at the clinic who needs to have her blood drawn for testing. Nurse Marge comes into the lab to inform Sara and Scott of the good news. "I've got one, Sara." She gives the information to the young investigator. "Room # 1."

"Thanks, we'll be right there." Sara acknowledges the message.

She and Scott leave the lab for exam room #1. Sara knocks on the door and the patient answers, "Come in." The woman is in her early 20's, with a slight build. She is at the clinic receiving her annual well woman exam and is getting and HIV and Syphilis test at the same time. "How are you doing?" Sara asks the young woman.

"I'm ok, the nurse said you were going to draw my blood."

"Yes, looks like I'll get one tube from you."

"Why's he here?" The patient motions to Scott.

Sara thinks for a second, "He's here to watch me."

"Are you new at this or something?"

"I've done this a couple of times so far." Sara is a little defensive, but also nervous. This is her first time drawing blood on a patient and she doesn't want to mess up. Sara had attended the phlebotomy training and drawn blood on Scott and Ann shortly after she was hired so she's familiar with the procedure, but is far from perfecting it. Scott advised her earlier that patients are for practice. That sounds a little cold, but the logic is sound. If she's going to get good at drawing blood in the field where there's no one watching and no back up, than she has to be able to do it in the clinic.

Sara sets up her blood draw materials on a small plastic stand that she places between herself and the patient. She puts on her gloves which are instantly filled with sweat. Her shaking hands manage to insert the needle into the vacationer. "Umm, which arm would you like for me to draw from?"

The woman, seeing how nervous the young public health worker is replies, "Neither, can he draw it?"

"It'll be ok, she's been well trained." Scott assures her.

Accepting, but not quite assured the patient thrusts her left arm towards Sara and rests it on the stand. Sara inspects the arm and locates a good spot to start. She applies the tourniquet, wipes the area with the alcohol pad, and inserts the needle into the patient's vein. "Ouch!" The woman cries out. The reaction further unsettles Sara causing her hands to shake even more.

Scott again assures the woman, "You'll be ok."

"But she's hurting me!"

"Take some deep breaths" Scott advises the young woman in a flat unsympathetic tone.

Sara has inserted the tube, but no blood is coming out. She pushes the needle in a little further, then a little further. The patient, who is in Scott's view overreacting, makes all kinds of wounded sounds. She tenses her muscles and is generally difficult to work with. Scott looks at the position of the needle. "I think you went through the vein" he tells Sara. "Pull it out and we'll try the other side."

Sara, who's becoming more nervous as the experience continues, withdraws the needle and blood streams down the patient's arm. "Take the tourniquet off" Scott suggests. "Crap!" Sara exclaims, and pulls the band off of the patient's arm stopping the flow of blood. "Here you go, you can use these." Scott hands Sara some cotton balls to clean up the blood. Sara's breathing is fast and her eyes are wide. Sweat has soaked her gloves and her heart is racing.

"Try the other arm." Scott tells the trainee.

The patient appearing distressed objects to the idea. "What?! Can't you do it?"

Scott assures her again, "You'll be alright."

Sara's panicked look does nothing to deter Scott. She and the patient exchange concerned looks at each other as Sara proceeds.

The second attempt is no more successful than the first was, though it appeared to be better tolerated. After the unsuccessful blood draw the woman was disinclined to allow Sara a third attempt. She seems irritated with Scott and prefers that they both leave the exam room. Scott and Sara comply with her wishes and leave the her alone in the room. The two investigators meet with Marge in the lab.

"You may have to use a butterfly on her." Scott suggests to the veteran nurse who looks at him with her head tilted to the side and arms crossed after he finishes stating the obvious. "Thanks" is all she says. Scott goes on, "Sara is going to hang out with you some this morning. Can you let her do all the blood draws for both you and Peggy please?" Marge looks at Sara, still visibly upset from her experience and remembers learning how to draw blood herself many years ago. "We'll watch after her, Scott." The nurse puts her arm around Sara to give her a little hug. It seems to help.

Scott returns to his office to review his notes on the investigation and write up what has occurred so far. Sara spends the rest of her morning sticking clinic patients, gaining experience, and getting to know the public health nurses who are the backbone of this organization.

Scott's phone rings while he is completing his vast amount of paperwork. "This is Scott."

"Hi Scott, Doctor Anderson at the ER, how are you?"

"I'm doing well, doctor, how are you?"

"Great," Dr. Anderson has worked off and on with Scott for the last couple of years. People with STDs will often go to the emergency room instead of the clinic so she and her staff have become very accustomed to working with these infections. State law requires doctors to notify the health department in cases of various diseases important to public health such as tuberculosis, West Nile, viral hepatitis, and in this case Syphilis. "I'm calling to report a positive Syphilis test."

Scott quickly grabs his pad and a pen from the cup on his desk. "Go ahead, I'm ready."

Dr. Anderson proceeds to give Scott the information she has on the patient she saw in her Emergency room, Chris Johnson. "Has she been notified of her results yet doctor?"

"Not yet, I was going to call her right after getting off the phone with you. She wasn't treated for Syphilis while she was here so I was going to make a referral to your clinic."

"That'll work out well. Let her know she can just walk in. We'll be open until five."

"Ok, and Scott."

"Yes?"

"She's pregnant."

A long pause emphasizes the seriousness of this news. "I think I'll call her if it's ok with you, doctor."

"That would be fine, let me know if you need anything, talk with you next time."

The line goes dead. Pregnant women and syphilis is the reason STD clinics were started in this country. The bacterium causes serious damage to the fetus while it is developing and can lead to serious deformities and death. Scott immediately picks up the phone and calls Chris.

"Hello?"

Grateful for an answer to his call, "Is Chris Johnson there please?" Scott's voice sounds stressed.

"Speaking, who is this?

"Chris, this is Scott at the health department." Scott confirms that he's talking with the right person then continues. "Your lab tests came in and we need to treat you for Syphilis today."

The patient is quiet for a moment. "I'll be right there." She hangs up the phone. Scott walks over to the registration counter. "Hey James, I've got a Chris Johnson coming in. Can you let me know when she gets here?" James nods and enters the woman's appointment into the clinic computer.

It takes Chris about a half hour to reach the clinic, but she arrives just before the staff are due to go to lunch. She is wearing pajama bottoms and a hooded sweat shirt and has a small child in tow. The child, about seven years old, is also in pajamas. James looks up at the pair and immediately recognizes the woman. Sandy looks at the mother and daughter as they walk into the clinic and wonders why the kid isn't in school. She shakes her head and looks down at her paperwork.

"Good morning Mrs. Johnson." James cheerfully greats the woman.

Ignoring the polite gesture, Chris informs James "I've got an appointment to see Scott."

"Yes ma'am. I'll get you checked in quickly and let him know you're here." James reports in the clinic computer that the patient has arrived and prints out some labels and inserts a few forms into her chart that he pulled earlier.

After completing the necessary paperwork James walks the chart back to Scott, who is sitting in his office and between phone calls. "She's here." James announces.

"Thanks James." Scott accepts the chart from James' outstretched hand and opens it. He quickly reviews the patient's history before bringing her back. "A couple of Chlamydia infections, a Gonorrhea, abnormal pap, she was treated three times as a contact to Gonorrhea. Her last syphilis test was 14 months ago, had a negative HIV at that time too." Scott talks out loud as he assesses. "It was just a matter of time before you got something major, Mrs. Johnson." Scott closes the chart and walks to the lobby and calls out, "Chris Johnson."

"I'm here!" the frightened woman stands and grasps the child's hand. Scott would prefer not to interview her while with the child and is thinking about how to separate them. He looks at his watch and thinks, "Why isn't that kid in school?" Scott walks back to exam room # 3 with the woman and the child. "Wait here for a moment, I'm going to get my coworker."

Scott walks down to Sara's office where she is again working on the training. He sees her reading on the computer again, the "Pink Snake" now situated on her desk. "How's the training coming?" Scott asks. Sara looks up, her expression greatly improved from the blood drawing incident "I'm almost done! I should be finished this afternoon. What's up?"

"We've got Mrs. Johnson here. She tested positive for Syphilis out of the ER." Scott reports.

Sara locks her computer and follows Scott to the exam room. On the way Scott asks her, "How was the blood drawing this morning?"

Sara seems relieved, "Much better. I got 7 of 10. Some of them were hard sticks though. The patients were dehydrated or overweight. That makes it hard to find the veins." Scott agrees "That it does. You'll find it in the field too. Get as good as you can. It may be the only opportunity some of these people have to receive a test." Sara nods in acknowledgment.

Scott knocks on the door and enters. Sara follows him inside the exam room where she sees a woman and a child waiting for them. Sara thinks, "Shouldn't that kid be in school?" but she dismisses the observation as soon as she has it. "Chris this is Sara, she's going to accompany us today.

"Did they tell you at the ER that your pregnancy test was positive?" Scott asks Chris while at the same time informing Sara of the situation. Sara instantly grasps the seriousness of this event.

"Ya, they told me. Said I have Gonorrhea too."

Scott nods in agreement, "They treated you for the Gonorrhea, and we are going to treat you for the Syphilis today. Hopefully we caught these infections in time before they harm your baby."

The mother appears concerned for the first time Scott's seen her. He's talked with her numerous times in the past but has not gotten much out of her. Now though, with the health of her unborn child at risk, she may be willing to talk. He looks at Sara who is showing genuine concern for the woman and her baby. The child grasps her mother tightly and appears intimidated by Scott. The woman herself is now very quiet.

"Sara, can you finish talking with the Mrs. Johnson please. I'll be in my office if you need me."

"Umm, sure" Sara accepts. She thinks, "This morning I've learned to draw blood, now I'm doing solo interviews with pregnant syphilis patients. Talk about getting thrown to the wolves." Scott steps out of the exam room # 3 and goes to exam room # 2 and sits against the adjoining wall. An unfortunate design flaw in the clinic allows people in the exam room over to listen in on what's being said. Scott suspects that his gender and familiarity with the patient may interfere with the interview. Allowing Sara to do it may be much more productive. Besides, Sara needs the experience. This investigation will help her to mature a great deal as a public health worker.

Sara conducts a good interview. She connects with Chris in a way that Scott never could. She is sympathetic, nonjudgmental, patient, and compassionate. The woman tells Sara about her husband Eddie "Red" Johnson, who she blames for giving her Gonorrhea. She also discloses to Sara that she has, on a few occasions, had sex with her husband's friend Grimy. The woman breaks down when she admits that she doesn't know whose baby she's carrying. Sara handles all of the drama and multiple angles of this case with professionalism. Chris doesn't remember seeing any sores or rashes on either of them. Sara educates Chris about the dangers of STD's especially while pregnant.

Scott goes to the employee lounge to locate a nurse willing to cut her lunch short to provide treatment. He finds Peggy sitting at the table enjoying a microwave meal of some sort of meat like substance, mashed potatoes and green beans. She's sipping on a diet soft drink. The nurse eyes Scott as he enters the lounge. "Hey Peggy, how's your lunch?"

Peggy swallows the diet soda in her mouth and answers in a grumpy tone, "What do you want Scott?"

"I need you to give a shot" Scott says politely getting right to the point. The nurse wipes her mouth and addresses the investigator who knows how much she values her lunch time.

"I knew I should have gone out to lunch." The nurse says half jokingly. "Take the bicillin out of the refrigerator and put it on the counter in the exam room and I'll be down in a min."

"Thank you Peggy, there's a special place in heaven for public health nurses." Scott says it jokingly, but has a very high regard for nurses who are willing to forgo decent pay and career progression to work in public health. It's not for everyone, but the lives they touch makes it well worth the sacrifices. Scott smiles at her and she shoos him away with a hand gesture.

Scott does as he was asked and gets the prefilled shots from the refrigerator in the lab and takes them to the exam room. He knocks and Sara opens the door. "How's it going?"

"Well, we were just finishing." Sara reports. Scott sets the medication down on the cabinet. "Peggy will be down shortly to administer the shots. We'll need you to wait around for a while after you get them."

"That's fine," Mrs. Johnson says. "Thank you."

Scott walks back to towards his office. James meets him in the hall. "Labs are in." James hands Scott a sealed manila envelope from the state lab. "Took long enough," Scott says under his breath. The state lab is very efficient, but when Scott is awaiting test results it feels like it takes forever. Scott sits down at his desk and opens the labs looking for one in particular. He locates it half way through the stack. "Negative" He reads on the report. "Peaches test is negative for Syphilis and HIV." He ponders the meaning of this test in context of the investigation. It's possible that she could have been infected by Lawrence or James and the infection is still too early to pick up by the lab, but she's not a source for either of them.

Scott calls Peaches to inform her of her test results. After hearing some unintelligible rap song for about 2 minutes Scott is forced to leave a vague voice message asking her to call him back. About three minutes later she does. "This is Scott." He recognizes her number from the caller ID. "Scott, this is Peaches, you called me?"

"Yes, we have your test results and I need you to come to the clinic so I can talk with you. Can you come down now?"

Peaches voice emanates concern about the upcoming conversation. She knows she was tested last week and also likely that there's been something going on among her group of associates. "I'll be right there." She says before getting off of the phone.

Scott sits back in his chair and thinks for a moment. He'll tell Peaches that she has a negative lab test, but also that she needs to be treated because that test might not pick up an early infection. But the question is how to do that without telling her that it's someone she's recently had sex with. "It's my job to maintain patient confidentiality, not keep patient's secrets." He concludes. "If she figures it out there's nothing I can do about it."

Scott looks at his watch; his doctor's appointment is coming up in about an hour. He's nervous about what might be wrong, but also knows much of it is out of his control. Scott looks over at the picture of his girls on the book case and smiles. They've gotten so big. It's amazing how time escapes and we lose touch with what's important. It's about balance. "I'm going to call them tonight and make an effort to spend more time before they grow up and it's too late." Scott finishes the self conversation more hopeful about the future and with a greater sense of well being.

Within only a few minutes Peaches arrives at the clinic. James calls back to Scott and Scott goes to the reception desk to meet her. "Thank you for coming in so quickly." Scott says to the young woman. "Come on back."

The two walk back to exam room #1 and Scott sits her down to explain what's going on.

"Your test results were negative," Scott informs her.

"Oh thank God! I thought you were going to tell me I had AIDS."

"Well here's the thing. I found out recently that you were exposed to Syphilis. Even though your test was negative, you could still have it if you were exposed recently." Peaches appears confused. "So I'm negative, but I could still have it? How's that work?"

Scott continues, "The test looks for an immune response and if you were recently infected your body may not have had time to develop that immune response yet. We are going to get some more blood from you today to run another test. We will also treat you today just in case you do have Syphilis."

Peaches still looks confused but she's accepting of the recommendation. "What's the treatment?"

"Penicillin. You'll get a couple of shots in your hips and it'll kill the bacteria if you have it. I'll go get the nurse and she'll be with you shortly" Scott leaves the exam room and finds Nurse Marge again. "Hey Marge…"

The nurse gives him the look again "Ya, I'll treat her. You're going to be late by the way."

Scott looks at his watch, another half hour passed and he didn't even realize it. "OK, I'm out of here. See you tomorrow."

Scott walks over to Sara's office and hands her his case notes along with the patient files. Sara's office door is open and she's sitting at her desk studying again. "Sara, these are my notes on the case and the patient files. I'm going to leave them with you while I'm out in case you need to reference something.

"Out?" Sara inquires.

"I've got an appointment this afternoon. I probably won't be back today, but will see you tomorrow morning."

"Oh, OK. Well good luck." Scott smiles and nods before leaving. He notices that sitting at her desk Sara reminds him of a younger version of Ann.

Scott goes back to his office briefly to pick up his bag and jacket. He also decides to send a quick e - mail to his boss to remind her that he'll be out. The computer is slow, probably because Scott is in a hurry. The e- mail is brief, "I'll be at an appointment this afternoon. Call if you need anything." Scott keeps his cell on him at all times and will answer it even if he's not at work. He closes down the computer and turns off the lights in the office before closing the door. As he passes the front desk he wishes Sandy and James a good afternoon before he leaves.

On his way to the doctor's office Scott calls both of his girls, who are in school, and leaves them a voice message. "Hi girls, this is your father. Hope you're having a good week. I was thinking about you and love you very much. Call me later when you get some time. Love you, bye."

Chapter 6

Sara finishes the basic training program and completes the final exam. It's no small task, but with that behind her she's able to focus on more than education. She picks up the pile of notes and cases that Scott left on her desk and searches through it for the next step to take. She finds two case reports that belong to patients who have not been contacted yet, Regan and Tiffany. James Jefferson said he had sex with both of them and that they attended the local high school. He didn't have any other information on them. Scott wrote the phone number to the high school on the case report form and attempted to call the school nurse but had to leave a message. Sara picks up the phone in an attempt to follow up with the school nurse. Finding these girls is critical, though Scott thinks they may be fictitious.

"School nurses office, Jennifer speaking."

"Hi Jennifer, my name is Sara and I work with Scott at the health department."

"Oh ya, how's Scott doing? He called me about a couple of girls and I haven't gotten back with him yet."

"He's doing well, but he's out this afternoon. He wanted me to follow up on some of these open cases so that's what I'm doing. Were you able to find info on these girls?"

The school nurse says in an apologetic voice, "No, I don't have anyone by that name and description dear. I'm sorry. Do you have a last name?"

"No, the guy who named them claimed he didn't know it. Thank you for looking though."

"I'll keep an eye out and if I come across any new information I'll let you know." The school nurse offers.

Sara appreciates the gesture, but realizes it's probably futile. Sara locates James' file and writes down his address and phone number on her note pad. She tries the number first hoping to set up an appointment to meet with him. The phone rings.

"What's up?" a man's voice booms from the other line.

"Is James Jefferson there please?" Sara asks.

"Who is this?"

"This is Sara at the clinic."

The phone goes dead. "Hello?" Sara calls. Soon a dial tone begins and she realizes that he hung up on her. Slightly offended Sara calls James back. The phone rings for a while, then the voice mail provides her the opportunity to enjoy a crass low quality rap recording before a voice is heard asking the caller to leave a message. She leaves one.

"James, this is Sara. One of our phones must have dropped the call, because we were disconnected. Please give me call back, I have important health information to discuss with you." She hangs up. Sara has no expectation that James will call her back, but she wants him to know that she won't just give up. Not when there are two young girls' lives at stake. She prepares a referral and gets directions to James' house so she can stop by this afternoon. Maybe she'll have better luck in person.

Sara return's to the interview notes. "Hmm, the next on my list is getting Red treated." She locates his number on the case report form and calls Red. She's fortunate that Red picks up. It's likely that he recognized the clinic's number and/or was told about the exposure and was expecting a call. He sounds very cordial this time.

"Hello." Red answers the call.

"Hi, is Mr. Eddie Johnson there please." Sara uses his legal name to emphasize the importance and validity of this call.

"That's me." Red replies, already knowing who is calling.

"Mr. Johnson, my name is Sara, we met at the clinic earlier. You've been exposed to syphilis and we need you to come back to the clinic to get treated. Can you come in now?" Asking him to come in now instead of making an appointment for later this afternoon, or even a day or two later emphasizes the serious nature of the condition.

"I'll be right there." Red replies.

"Ok, the front desk will expect you, thanks." Sara hangs up the phone and calls the front desk. "This is Sandy."

"Hi Sandy, Sara. Mr. Eddie Johnson is coming to the clinic now. Can you check him in and let me know when he arrives please?"

"Ok." Sandy responds.

Sara recalls that Scott makes it a point to always walk to the desk and communicate with the administrative assistants. He does the same thing with the clinic nurses. Sara finds this approach terribly inefficient. She explains it to herself, "It's probably just a generational gap thing. Older workers are just not as used to communicating with technology as the younger more tech savvy generation is." The reality is that Scott uses interpersonal communication to improve the working relationships with people. He finds that even though face to face communication takes longer, the relationships it builds improves patient care. Plus, it gives him a chance to stretch his legs.

Sara's phone rings and she answers. "Sara, your patient is here."

"Ok, thank you. I'll be up shortly." The phone goes dead. Sara again gathers her interview kit and proceeds to the front desk to retrieve Red. She meets him at the front desk. He's elected not to sit in the waiting area. Eddie is agitated. His emotional balance seems off, in fact he's angrier than what Sara would expect. "Hi Mr. Johnson, come on back please." His gait is fast and powerful. His breathing is hard and eyes are very intent.

Sara is a little concerned about him becoming violent, but his anger doesn't seem to be directed at her. She opens the exam room door and he walks in and sits down.

"What's wrong?" Sara inquires.

"Chris told me she's been fuck'n Grimy." He discloses. "She even had my girl over there."

"Your girl?" Sara inquires.

"Ya, my daughter." Eddie elaborates. "That aint no place for a kid."

Sara agrees. Not much of a place for adults.

"What did Chris tell you about what's going on?" Sara attempts to redirect and gain some insight for her investigation.

"She told me she got Syphilis from Grimy and that I need to come down here to get checked out. This is some bull shit!" Red pounds his hand against his legs.

"Well, we are going to get you taken care of today. You'll get a couple of shots that'll get ride of the Syphilis if you do have it." Sara again attempts to redirect him. Her attempts are not effective. Red seems very focused on his angry feelings towards Grimy and Chris.

"If that motha fuck'r touched my girl I'm going to kill him!"

Sara pauses for a moment. The horrific thought hadn't occurred to her and now that it does she's stunned and loses track of her investigation.

"Umm, I'm going to get the nurse so they can get some blood from you and get your shots. I'll be right back." Sara excuses herself and leaves the exam room. She recalls seeing the little girl yesterday with the pajama bottoms and Sesame Street t shirt. She was wearing ponytails and had big brown eyes. She recalls how the girl hid behind her mother and wanted nothing to do with Scott. She should have been in school…but she wasn't. Sara feels a rush of unexplainable emotion well up in her chest that makes it difficult to breathe. Her hands shake as she thinks about that child in the filthy crack house. Sara tries to regain her senses. "Think dammit. What's the next step?" Her first instinct is to call the police, but she remembers

Scott telling patients that the disease investigators don't work with the police. Fortunately Ann passes Sara in the hall and sees that she is distressed.

"Sara, are you ok." Ann stops and talks with the young investigator.

Sara, now remembering Ann's open door policy responds. "Do you have a minute?"

Concerned, Ann touches Sara's shoulder. "Of course, come to my office." The two climb the stairs. Sara's mind is racing. She's not even sure how to explain what she's thinking.

Ann sits at her desk and Sara across from her. "What's going on?" Ann asks her new employee.

"Do you remember the drug dealer Lawrence, he goes by Grimy?"

"Yes, he's part of your Syphilis investigation." Ann pauses to allow Sara to continue.

"He may have exposed a little girl."

"How little?" Ann has been a nurse for a couple of decades and has some experience with child sex offenders; still the information is disturbing to a veteran public health nurse.

"Seven." Sara says with conviction. The child's frightened face flashes yet again in her mind.

Ann sits back in her chair and folds her hands. "How do you know?"

Sara admits, "I don't. The father is in the exam room and brought it up as a possibility, but it makes sense."

Ann nods, "OK, so you don't know anything yet. Try to relax. When Scott gets back we'll investigate and figure things out."

Sara, still having a terrible feeling realizes that Ann is right. She still feels compelled to do something though. "Scott won't be back until tomorrow. What can we do about this now?"

Ann tries to defuse some of Sara's anxiety. "The mother isn't here right?" Sara nods. "The child isn't here either?" Again Sara agrees. "The only thing you know is that the father, who's not entirely reputable, is saying that something might have happened?" Sara feels a little trapped. Her desire to do something and her ability are at odds. She hates the idea, but accepts that she'll have to wait. "Hmm," she thinks to herself, "Maybe."

"Thank you Ann, I'll keep you up to date on any important developments." Sara stands. Ann looks at her, noting the change in emotion. "OK Sara, we'll talk later." Sara leaves Ann's office and walks downstairs.

Sara finds Marge waylaid at the lab by the courier. Marge is trying to get back to the patient in her exam room, but is also trying to make sure that all of the specimens are ready for him to take to the state lab.

"Hi Marge, are you busy?" Sara asks seeing that the clinic nurse is clearly preoccupied.

"Yes Sara, I've got these specimens that need to go out and a patient waiting for me. What do you need?

"When you get some time Eddy is in the room and needs to get treated and tested again. Thank you." Sara smiles at the nurse who responds with a frustrated scowl. Sara returns to her office and picks up the phone. "This is Scott,"

"Scott, I know you're busy but I need to talk with you. Are you coming back this afternoon?" Sara realized by watching Scott work that if she makes patient care an urgency people are much more likely to act quickly and properly. "Ya, Hopefully I'll be done in the next hour or so."

"Great, see you then." Sara hangs up.

After some time Marge meets with Red in the exam room. He's been there for maybe twenty minutes, but sufficient time has passed to allow him to calm down some. "Hi Eddy, you're back soon." Marge comment is directed to his earlier visit for Gonorrhea treatment. "Ya, that bitch gave me Syphilis this time. The nurse plays devil's advocate with him "How do you know it's her and not you?"

"Oh I know, she got caught this time."

The nurse prepares the medication for Red, "All I'm saying is that if you're having sex with more than one person you really can't know where you got infected from." The information marinates with Red, but he's still dedicated to the idea that Chris infected him. "OK, let me see those cheeks."

"Ouch!" Sara hears the cry from down the hall. She wants to talk with him before he leaves. The time he has to wait after getting the shots provides a perfect opportunity for her to re-interview him. She prepares some questions for Red and writes them on her pad before going to the exam room.

Sara enters the room where Red is having his blood drawn by the nurse. "Hi again Red, how are you?"

"Pissed off and sore. How are you?" He replies facetiously.

"Better now. I'm glad we got you taken care of. Red, I have some more questions for you. Who have you had sex with over the last year?"

"Com'on! I already answered this shit. How many times you gon'a ask me the same questions?" Red begins to get agitated again.

"OK, let's talk about other people. You said that Chris is having sex with Grimy, who else is she having sex with?"

"Prob'ly every motha fuck'r out there." Red waves his hand to suggest outside.

"OK, what are their names? I'm going to need to find them so that we can get them tested and treated too." Sara gets the impression that Red doesn't know anyone other than Lawrence because the accusation was too vague.

"I dun'o, you got to ask her."

"OK, we'll follow up with her. What about Grimy. Who else is he having sex with?" This is the question that Sara really wanted to ask. She knows that Red and Grimy are friends and Red likely knows some of Grimy's other partners. Now that Red is upset with Grimy, he may be willing to provide information that previously he wasn't willing to.

"Shit, that motha fucka will do anything that sit still long enough." Red speaks ill of his former friend. Red thinks of all of the women who have come and gone from Grimy's place. Some of them they had sex with at the same time. He shakes his head, lamenting the way things worked out for him.

"Look, Grimy pays bit.. I mean women for pussy. Sometime it be cash, sometime rock. My girl Chris used to smoke a lot, but she got off that shit." He hangs his head again and shakes it. "Thought she got off it when we had our last kid."

"I duno most of em. Shit, can't tell you bout non of em. The main girl that hang around is Angela. She stay at Grimy's place so you can find her there. I seen't this girl Rose over there. Grimy do'n her, but I duno where she at." Red provides descriptions of Angela and Rose. Sara recognizes them from earlier on in the investigation. "That's it." Red shakes his head.

Sara appreciates his cooperation. She can almost sense that he's turned a corner in his life. "Thank you, you've been a great help."

"Ya, well I'm out't. You be good. Hope I never hear from you again." Red's statement is partially a joke. He means that he doesn't want to come back to the STD clinic. Sara appreciates the goal and reciprocates. "Good luck to you Red." As he turns to leave Sara is grabbed by the sense that she should capitalize on this opportunity. "Hey Eddie?"

Eddie stops, anticipating more talking about partners or something else that he didn't want to discuss. "What's up?"

"I'd like for you to talk with our social worker before you go. I think he can help you."

Eddie doesn't appear enthusiastic about the idea. Social workers are not highly regarded in his social circles. "What fo?"

"He may have some ideas to help you take your life in the direction you want it to go in. It won't take long and if you want to stop talking to him at any time you can." It might be Sara's insistence or her concern for him that changes Eddie's mind about seeing the social worker. He hasn't had many people care about him in his life and this one seems to want to help. Eddie does want his life to improve. He's tired of getting infected, he's tired of the violence, and he wants his kids to have more than he did. But he doesn't know how to get the life that he wants.

"I guess, I'll hear him out."

Sara smiles at him. "I'll get him now." Sara arranges for Eddie to see the clinic social worker and walks Eddie to his office.

Scott returns to the clinic from his doctor's appointment. The hour is late and the clinic will be closing in the next few minutes. The staff at the front desk have already closed the computers down, Sandy is filing the patient charts from the afternoon rush, while James is walking the halls making sure the patients are gone, the lights are off, and the doors to the offices are closed and locked. They complete their duties with grand efficiency.

Scott walks past the check in desk, past his office, and to Sara's office where he finds her mulling over case report forms and notes, oblivious to the late hour. "Hi Sara, what's going on?"

Sara's had some time to think about all that's transpired and has calmed somewhat. But she's still plenty upset about the child she perceives is in danger. "How was the doctor's visit?"

"It was fine, just ran some tests." Scott isn't one to belabor his medical concerns. Besides, he doesn't know anything yet.

"Red was back this afternoon. I called him in to get him treated and when I cluster interviewed him he linked Lawrence with Rose." She gives Scott the good news.

"That's great." Scott replies. He was pretty sure the two outbreaks were linked. He just wishes Sara would have waited till morning to tell him that. "Well we'll be back at it again tomorrow. Have a good night." Scott attempts to leave.

"Scott," Sara calls him back. "There's more." Hearing her tone Scott takes off his jacket and has a seat in Sara's office across the desk from her. He gets a sense of deja vu since the position is the same as when he is in Ann's office. His mind wanders a little, wondering why Sara and Ann have people sit across the desk from them and he has people sit at the side of his desk. Hmm, and Sara's desk is bigger than his. "Scott," Sara calls him again and he snaps back to the here and now. "Yes,"

"Lawrence might have exposed Chris's little girl." Sara knows Scott will have the answer to solve this important problem.

Scott's initial reaction is that of skepticism. He hears wild accusations on a regular basis. But, he remembers seeing the child in the clinic and getting the feeling that something was very wrong. Not just like her mother and father are crack addicts and keep her out of school sort of wrong, but that there was something else. With all of the science and training, and procedures, and experience that Scott has at this job, sometimes intuition is what makes the difference.

"What makes you think that?" Scott wants all of the information before he makes any assessments regarding the validity of a claim.

"Red mentioned that it was possible."

"Red mentioned that it's possible?" Scott repeated. "Sara, that's pretty weak."

"I know it is, but we've got to do something."

"We will, absolutely." Scott asserts.

"Really?!" Sara's hopes are raised.

"Of course, we'll get her tested." Scott continues

"Tested? That's it?" That was not the intervention that Sara had hoped for.

"Well, and treated if need be. I'll call her pediatrician and arrange it first thing in the morning."

"You're not going to call the police, social services, or somebody?"

"No, you and I are not mandatory reporters. Nurses, Doctors, and social workers are required to report child abuse if they suspect it. Not us."

Now outraged, Sara's passion is rekindled "So if we know that a person is abusing a child we won't report it?!"

"No, that's not what we do."

"That's unacceptable! How can you be ok with letting children get abused and do nothing."

"I didn't say we would do nothing. We're going to get her tested. And if she's positive we'll get her treated."

"I absolutely can not believe what I am hearing!" Sara, now completely astonished. Her respect for Scott as a caring human being, a decent human being is gone. She doesn't know how he could be so cold. What is it about this job that allows him to think this is ok? Maybe he's worked so hard to "understand" these people that he's lost his humanity, his decency, his common sense. She is appalled and speechless.

Scott sees Sara is in conflict and senses she is upset with him. He's been doing this so long maybe he's become a little insensitive.

"Sara," he says in a calm voice. She doesn't look at him. "No matter what you think about the actions of our patients, they have to trust us. Trust is the only tool we have to get them to talk with us. If they think for a minute that we will take the information they give us and tell the authorities that trust is out the door. We will not be able to find people who've been exposed, we won't be able to educate, and we won't be able to stop the spread of disease. We are the only ones who do what we do. And if we can't intervene in the disease process it will spread throughout the community, people will get sick and die. That's how important our job is."

Sara listens to Scott; she's upset but knows on some level that what he's saying makes sense. Scott continues, "We look at the big picture. Disease intervention is about the health of the community, not an individual. That's why we contact people, that's why we treat people. The diseases we work with can infect and affect a population if it's not stopped. You don't see disease investigators running around trying to stop diabetes, obesity, or smoking. Why? Because those conditions affect individuals. There's no spread.

"So we are going to get her tested and treated and that's it?" Sara still hopeful that Scott will impress her with some strategy to get justice.

Scott thinks about it for a long moment. They don't interview children for good reason. Children with STDs are victims of sexual abuse and that's a matter for social services, the police, and the courts.

"We are not going to report this to child welfare or the police, Sara." Scott affirms. "It's not our job. I won't sacrifice our credibility for one person."

Sara slumps. It's a hard pill to swallow and she doesn't know if she can continue to do this job if it means letting child molesters go free.

Scott doesn't care for people who harm children either, and while he vows to play by the rules and do what's best, he's not above going around them from time to time.

"Feel like some dinner?" Scott asks Sara.

"No, I feel sick." Sara expresses her displeasure with the situation and directs it at Scott.

"Come on, a grande burrito and a margarita will improve your disposition. I'm buying."

Sara begrudgingly accepts. The two put on their jackets and leave her office. The clinic hallway is dark save the emergency lights. The coworkers walk down the long dark hall to the exit and into the parking lot. The smell of Mexican food is heavy in the air. The air is cold and it's already getting dark. The last remnants of sunlight leave pink and orange designs across the western sky. Sara feels her stomach rumble; she is hungry. Sara thinks "Come to think of it I haven't eaten since breakfast." Scott and Sara make their way across the parking lot to the restaurant.

The restaurant has large wooden doors with handles in the shape of tamales. The colors are vibrant and the restaurant is filled with happy inebriated people talking loudly to be heard over each other and the festive background music. A short, but wide man approaches the two. He is wearing a shirt with the restaurant logo, a large tamale, a taco, and a burrito on it. They appear to be chasing a margarita but it's hard to make out. "Two?" the server asks Scott. "Three" Scott replies. He turns to Sara and talks close to her ear. "This is date night for Patty and I; she'll join us shortly."

Sara yells over the noise of the crowd so Scott can hear her. "Who's Patty?"

Scott laughs, "I do have a life."

"Are you sure I'm not in the way? I don't want to interrupt your date night."

"It's fine. She wants to meet you." Scott reassures Sara.

The server motions for the two of them to follow him and seats them at a booth about half way down the long row of seats. The benches are carved with characters and the tables have vivid laminated posters depicting what Sara believes to be culturally significant images.

The waiter brings the customary chips, salsa, and water and asks for a drink order.

"We'll take two margaritas please." Scott orders for both of them.

Scott sits in the bench facing the entrance so he can see Patty when she comes in. Not long after he put in the drink order, he sees her. She's off from a long day of work, but it doesn't show. She appears vibrant and fresh. Scott waves at her and she walks towards the table where the investigators are sitting.

Scott stands and greets Patty with a kiss and a hug. He takes her coat and lays it next to his on the bench. Patty sits on the bench first then Scott next to her. "Patty this is Sara, Sara this is my beautiful girlfriends and wonderful all around person, and fabulous nurse Patty." Patty cuts her eyes at Scott for the embellished introduction and reaches across the table to shake hands with Sara. "Nice to meet you." She says with a smile. "Scott's told me a lot about you."

"Really? That's nice." Sara is still taken off guard. Scott's told her nothing about Patty, but then again, Sara doesn't know much about Scott at all outside of work.

"What has he said?" Sara asks Patty causing Scott to react surprised by the question, and a little embarrassed.

Patty looks at Scott smiling as she tortures him by this display of humiliation. "He said you are very smart and that you're catching onto the job much faster than he did. He said you are ambitious, professional, and how did you put it again?" Patty looks at Scott, who is partially covering his face with his hands in an attempt to ignore the conversation.

"How did I put what?" Scott surrenders to the questioning.

"What did you say she would end up doing?" Patty jogs his memory.

"Oh look, chips" Scott evades the question and stuffs his mouth with tortilla chips so he can't possibly speak.

"That's so juvenile." Patty shakes her head as she looks at him. She turns her attention towards Sara, "He thinks very highly of you and that you have a very bright future in public health."

Sara intentionally acts overly sappy and responds to Scott "Awwww, you're so sweet, thank you soooo much." She and Patty laugh and the waiter brings the Margaritas. Scott gives his to Patty and orders another.

The three of them enjoy an evening of talking and joking, mostly at Scott's expense. The food is good, the margaritas are good, and the company is great. A couple of hours later Sara looks at her watch. "I've got to get home and let my dog out. Poor thing will have her legs crossed."

"It was nice to meet you Sara," Patty shakes her hand across the table.

"Likewise," Sara returns the gesture and puts on her jacket. "Good night Scott, see you in the morning."

"Good night Sara, be safe." Scott replies.

Sara leaves the restaurant which has lost much of its business to the late hour. The staff are beginning to put the chairs on the tables and have mop buckets and swabs at the ready to complete their evenings tasks. Scott and Patty get up from the bench. Scott helps Patty put on her jacket before putting on his own and they walk to the register check in hand.

"This was fun, we'll have to do it again soon." Scott comments to his girlfriend who nods in agreement.

"I like her a lot." Patty tells Scott. "You can just tell that she's a good caring person."

"Yes, but in this business that can be both an asset and a liability." Scott cautions. "We have to care, but if we get emotionally involved in what's going on with the patients it will burn us out and we'll be no good to anyone."

Being a nurse for many years Patty understands what Scott's saying and agrees. Balancing how much emotion to put into the job is difficult and can only be learned by experience. "She'll be fine Scott."

"Ya, I think so." The two leave the restaurant. Scott walks Patty to her car and opens the door. "Following me home?" He asks with a smile.

"Of course." Patty returns the smile. The couple kiss and Scott hugs her before they leave.

Chapter 7

Sara arrives at the clinic at about a quarter till eight after a very full stomach led her to a good night's sleep. "Good morning," Sara greets the administrative staff. They are getting the clinic ready to see patients shortly. Sara walks back towards the offices and sees Scott's light on and door open.

"How's your morning Scott?" Sara sounds much better than she did the afternoon before.

"I'm good, today is going to be a good day." Scott asserts with confidence.

"Oh ya? Why do you say that?"

"Because today we are going to stop the spread of disease." Scott's tone could be taken as comical, but there is conviction behind his words. Sara looks at him inquisitively for a moment before thinking to herself, "He actually believes that."

Sara follows up her last questions "So what's on the list?"

Scott looks over his notes and identifies some priority cases that need intervention. "Got to get Rose and bring her into the clinic for treatment and testing. I know she's been avoiding your calls, but if you show up at her house again we may have more luck. In the mean time I'm going to do some digging around and see if I can't find some useful information to help with the case we talked about last night."

The last statement piqued Sara's curiosity, but she doesn't inquire about it. Instead she complies with

Scott's instructions. "OK, I'll be back shortly." Scott hands Sara Rose's information and she leaves the clinic in search of Rose Drake and the truth.

Sara recalls the house, but not exactly how to get there. She uses the Google map to help guide her towards the location, but reading the printed map and navigating the car simultaneously proves to be difficult, and a little dangerous. "I need to invest in a GPS" Sara mutters.

She does arrive safely at the location. She notices that the same red Impala is parked in the drive of the one story blue house. Sara parks a couple of houses before the target to watch it for signs of people being home prior to approaching. She is irritated that this patient lied to her about her partners. Sara could have gotten her treated earlier if she had the correct information, but now, it's possible that more people could have been exposed.

Leaving her car and approaching the house slowly, ever watching for movement, Sara moves towards the front door. She hears the dog barking inside, then stop barking. She half smiles to herself. "Not going to work this time Ms. Drake." Sara knocks loudly on the door. No answer. She waits a little while but still nothing. Sara knocks again, but again no answer.

The quandary motivates Sara towards innovation. Sara knocks again very loudly and follows it up by saying in a loud voice, "Rose Drake! This is Sara! We talked a couple of days ago! It's really important that I talk with you again!"

The angry woman opens the door, "What do you want?!"

"You have syphilis, we need to get you treated." The sudden news seems to defuse the woman. She agrees to follow Sara to the health department for treatment.

Sara walks into Scott's office. "She's here." Sara says with pride.

"Good job. How did you get her?" Scott remembers having some difficulty getting this woman to come to the door.

"I knocked on the door and asked for her." Sara states, not sure if banging and yelling would be acceptable. But then again, it is Scott she's talking to.

"Whatever works." Scott validates her efforts.

"You're just in time. I did some digging this morning and found the pediatrician who takes care of Chris's children. Her name is Dr. Frea Hodge out of the Southland Pediatric Clinic."

Sara holds her breath. "How did you find that?"

"I'll show you later, but for now we need to call so that we can get the child tested."

Scott uses the speaker phone and calls the pediatric clinic. "Hi, may I speak with Dr. Hodge or her nurse please, this is Scott from the health department." Scott winks at Sara and she smiles. Dr. Hodges nurse picks up the call, "Hi Scott, this is Linda, what's up?" Like many health care providers, Scott has worked with this nurse on many occasions.

"Hay Linda, I'm calling about Katherine Johnson, she's Chris and Eddie's child."

"OK," the nurse's expression gives away that she knows something more than she's let on. The nurse is limited by confidentiality as far as what she can tell Scott. "What about her?"

"We think she may have been exposed to Syphilis, and possibly gonorrhea." Scott is direct with his communication.

"Oh Lord, that doesn't surprise me. That poor child."

"Can you have the Dr. bring her in for syphilis testing?"

"Yes of course. Did you contact child welfare?"

"No, I can't contact them."

"Oh, OK." The nurse sounds disappointed that Scott wouldn't make the call to the authorities.

"Thanks Linda, we'll be in touch soon." Scott terminates the call.

"I thought you said we couldn't report?" Sara isn't arguing the act, she just wants to understand Scott's change of heart.

"I said that we don't report and I meant it. We can't tell police or report to child welfare. We are not mandatory reporters...but nurses are."

"She asked you to report." Sara points out.

"Ya, she doesn't want to report her patient's is all, but she will. Especially since we called her. Now we get to call Chris."

Scott again uses the speaker phone. The phone rings once and is picked up, "This is Chris." She likely recognized the clinic number again.

"Chris this is Scott from the clinic. We need to you take your daughter to her pediatrician for testing. She was named in the investigation and needs to be tested." Scott again bluntly stating fact brings about dead silence. Scott can't bring the child into the health department for testing or treatment because the clinic doesn't see children under the age of 12. Otherwise he would handle the patient care in house.

Chris's mind is racing and she considers all of the possibilities. She feels trapped. "OK" is all she can manage to reply.

"Good, they are expecting you. Please head over there now."

Chris agrees and the phone goes dead. "OK, we'll see what happens." Scott will get the child tested one way or another. That's his job. If the mother refuses than the doctor's office will contact social services and they'll intercede.

"Go check on your patient, make sure she gets taken care of. You might want to talk with her again, see who else she isn't telling us about." Scott suggests to Sara who is sitting in the chair trying to take in everything that just happened.

"Yes Sir." Sara salutes Scott in a friendly mocking manor. She leaves the office in search of Rose.

***

While Scott is completing his paperwork for the syphilis investigation his desk phone rings. The caller ID informs Scott that the call is coming from the Clear Lake Clinic, his doctor's office. "This is Scott."

"Hi Scott, this is Debbie at Dr. Stone's office. How are you?"

Scott hears the strain in Debbie's voice. She is usually so upbeat and cheerful. "I don't know,"

Scott says, concern welling up inside of his gut, "How am I?"

Realizing her previous tone conveyed more information that she had intended, Debbie's voice becomes even more dire. "Scott, we need you to come in."

For a moment Scott realizes how his patients must feel when he contacts them. He finds himself responding in a very similar way. "I'll be right there."

"OK, I'll let the Dr. know" the sympathetic voice does nothing to reassure Scott who fears the worst.

When Scott arrives at the doctor's office he is immediately brought into the exam room and asked to wait for a moment. Dr. Stone comes into the exam room after a few short moments with a somber look. "Scott, there's no easy way to put this. The cancer has returned. This time it's moved to your liver." The doctor goes on to say that he isn't sure if treatments will be effective at this stage. There are some things that they'll try, but the somber practitioner advises Scott to take some time off and get his affairs in order. Scott feels like he was hit by a sledge hammer. He doesn't feel like he's done living, and yet, he is. Many thoughts race through his mind, but at the forefront the more immediate question is how will he tell his girls. And how is Peggy going to take this news. "I'm going to make a referral for you to see a psychiatrist in addition to the oncologist you saw last time. They are going to help you through this. I'm Sorry Scott, I know this is a tough one to take."

Scott agrees, death is a tough one to take. Maybe he should have found a doctor with better bedside manner. Scott tells himself that he'll have to remember that for next time. The dry joke lightens his mood slightly. Scott leaves Dr. Stone's office and says good bye to Debbie. She's been a great nurse. He somberly leaves the office and returns to his car. Everything seems to be happening in slow motion since he heard the news of his impending, premature in his opinion, demise.

Scott calls Ann on his cell while walking to his car. The sun seems brighter, but the cold wind sends chills through his body. He lifts the collar on his jacket to shield himself, at least a little, from the wind. Ann answers, "Hi Scott, how did the doctor's appointment go?" The fact that Scott is calling her right after the appointment is not a good sign to her.

Scott fumbles for words for a moment; the lengthy pause does nothing to alleviate Ann's concerns. "It's not good. The cancer has returned and spread." Ann doesn't respond verbally, but Scott can only imagine how she is taking the news. They share the long silence in understanding friendship. The emptiness conveys more than words ever could. "Hey, I'm going to take the rest of the afternoon off. I'll come by in the morning so we can talk."

Ann is choked up, but maintains her composure. "OK Scott" she manages to force the words past her tightened throat. "I'm sorry." Scott hangs up and proceeds towards his car. It seems to have gotten colder since he left the building. Cold wet flakes land on his face. Shocked by the sensation, Scott looks up to the sky and witnesses the first flakes of winter fluttering down. They gently glide to the surface of his car and his jacket where they melt into tiny drops of water. Scott watches for a while. He takes in all of the cool air into his lungs and the bright light onto his face.

Scott drives towards the hospital. He is in need of company and can think of no one he'd rather be with right now that Patty. He calls her cell before reaching the hospital and the call goes right to voice mail. The customary message plays and requests that a message be left. "Hi Patty, I was in the neighborhood and wanted to know if you wanted to meet for coffee in the hospital cafeteria on a break. I'll head over there, umm… just call me back or meet me down there. Love you," Scott hangs up. He reaches the hospital and after driving around for a few minutes locates a parking spot in the visitors lot. Thankfully the parking lot is covered, because the snow is coming down harder now and beginning to settle on the street and walkways. Leaving his car, Scott walks towards the main entrance to the hospital. Near the front he sees a couple of patients in wheel chairs accompanied by hospital staff. One is a woman with a small bundle in her arms. The package of blankets is entirely covered and held close to her chest. And the other is an older women, perhaps in her 70s. She is dressed warmly for her exit from the hospital. The old woman admires the young mother. A large smile dominates her wrinkled face. Scott can't help but stare at the package, even though no child can be seen through the blankets. Babies carry with them the hopes of so many. Their lives are a canvas that can become a masterpiece, or a disaster. In Scott's experience they usually fall somewhere in the middle. He reflects on his one life wondering where it will fall on the spectrum.

A red Chevy Lumina pulls into the circular drive designated for patient loading. The young man who's driving, leaps out of the car and rushes to the passenger side where he opens the back door. He produces a plastic infant car seat and approaches the young mother. She gently lays the baby in the seat ensuring that every part of the infant is covered. After the newborn is strapped to the seat the young man whisks the child away and places the baby in the back seat of the car. He shuts the door and returns to the mother. Like a gentleman he helps her stand from the wheel chair and the couple smiles and says good bye to the hospital staff who has been helping them. The man opens the passenger side front door. The young mother declines and walks to the other side of the car and climbs into the back seat with the child. Scott laughs and says to himself "Must be a first child." The old woman never takes her eyes off of the couple as they pull away.

Scott stands and watches for a while. He hasn't heard from Patty and isn't in a hurry to loiter around the hospital lunchroom. The old woman is still brimming from her experience with seeing the baby and the mother. Soon, her ride pulls into the circular drive. The maroon Oldsmobile parks in front of the entrance and an old man slowly climbs from the driver's seat. He hobbles around the car to the woman waiting him. She is unsteady as she rises from the chair and he grasps her arm to help. They hug and kiss briefly before turning from the hospital worker who unlocks the brakes and returns inside with the chair.

Scott's eyes well up, but he forbids them from forming tears. He realizes that he and Patty will not have a chance to be that old couple and his chest tightens. The man helps his bride into the car before returning to his side. The old woman smiles at Scott as they pull away. Scott takes a few deep cold breaths and clears his eyes before going into the hospital's reception area. The large sectioned doors turn slowly counter clockwise forcing Scott to slow the pace of his walk considerably. Once inside he finds himself standing at the beginning of a very large reception room. At his right side is a line of wheel chairs. To his left are rows of soft chairs and benches that face an information desk which is staffed by an older man and woman, presumably volunteers, and a younger high school aged girl in a red and white striped shirt. "Good afternoon sir," the girl says to Scott. He's been in the hospital hundreds of times, but his slow progress through the room and his tourist appearance lead the girl to believe that Scott is in need of direction. "Can I help you find something?" she continues.

Scott was a little startled by the interaction. The young lady's voice snapped him out of his trance like state and he responds. "No, thank you. I'm going to the cafeteria."

The girl, believing that Scott does in fact need assistance, proceeds to describe how Scott can best reach his desired destination. "If you take a right at the wall and follow the hallway down past the gift shop, the cafeteria will be on your left." She provides these directions with a warm smile indicating her happiness to assist Scott. Scott avoids the temptation to act confused and have her repeat the directions a few times, though that would have been funny. He instead thanks the young lady for her help and proceeds down the hall.

As soon as he reaches the T intersection, Scott catches the scent of taco meat and French fries doubtless, left over from the facility's lunch. The grease smells heavenly, and Scott is a little hungry. The morbid thought that nothing he eats now will kill him enters his mind. Scott follows his olfactory senses towards the dining hall. As promised he passes the gift shop that is cluttered with bright colored over priced knickknacks, balloons, stuffed animals, flowers, candies, and reading material. He peers in for a moment and sees a staff woman working behind the register, but no customers are in the shop. He proceeds to his destination a short distance away.

The cafeteria is a very large space with hard chairs and large tables. The walls are painted stone and the floors are white tile. The dining part is sectioned off by stainless steel food preparation counters. The lunch rush has passed and now the employees are seen cleaning and talking. The mood is light in the dining hall. Scott approaches the line and requests something to eat. "May I have a couple of tacos and fries with a large coffee…oh and some water." The young man behind the counter assembles Scott's order on a plate and hands it to him on a tray. "The coffee is on the counter at the end of the fountain drinks, sir." Scott accepts the tray; the food doesn't look as good as it smells, but the proximity makes his stomach growl.

Scott finds a seat facing the entrance way to the cafeteria and sets his tray on one of the long tables. Leaving his meal to cool by itself, Scott crosses the room to the coffee station. The three selections take him a little while to figure out. They are not labeled well, but after some time the investigator determines that one is dark roast, another is a Caribbean blend, and the other is decaf. The idea of decaf coffee still perplexes Scott. He looks at the container with disdain and selects the dark roast. After adding a couple sugars and some cream, Scott returns to his seat. Not long after he sits down Patty walks into the cafeteria. She's beautiful in her work scrubs and quickly done hair with no makeup. Scott smiles at her and lifts his cup. Patty, unaccustomed to Scott stopping by her work and knowing that he met with the doctor today appears worried. She quickly walks over to his table and they hug briefly before she sits across from him.

Scott greets her as usual probably because it's familiar ground and he doesn't know how to tell her what's going on. "Do you want some coffee?" Scott offers. Peggy declines "No, thank you. How did your visit with the doctor go?" Peggy, not one to mince words gets to the point immediately. Scott should have expected this approach. He's known Peggy for years and she doesn't want to sit in suspense. She wants to know what's going on so she can address it, fix it. But there's no fixing this.

Scott's voice softens and he takes Peggy's hands in his. Her eyes are wide and her face betrays her scared feelings. "My cancer returned." Peggy is stunned, but at the same time expected the news. The reaction makes for a disruptive emotional paradox. "Oh Scott, I'm so sorry." She grasps his hands and holds them next to her face. Tears stream down her cheeks. After she gives herself a moment to grieve the news she looks at Scott's eyes and assures him "We'll get through this." Scott nods, saving the rest of the bad news for another time. Right now, they enjoy the ten minutes they have together while Peggy is on break. The couple spends the next few minutes talking about testing and treatment. Peggy is a problem solver and she won't rest till she's found a solution. Scott very much appreciates her support. He doesn't want to hurt her, but he loves her and will enjoy her company for as long as he can.

Peggy's watch alarm sounds indicating the end of her break. "I've got to get back to work, but we'll get together tonight." The statement is not phrased as a question. Scott holds Peggy in his arms tightly and kisses her good bye. "OK, see you tonight," he replies. She walks to the exit turning just before walking out of site and waves. Then she's gone, and Scott is alone in the cafeteria.

He adjusts in his chair. His tacos and fries are now cold. It's inconsequential because he's lost his appetite. Scott takes a sip of his coffee, which he finds is also cold. He sits back in his seat and listens to the sounds of the hospital. People passing in the halls, the kitchen workers talking, and the music over the communication system all blend together in a harmonious atmosphere.

Scott finishes his cold coffee and leaves the hospital. On the way home he stops by the liquor store and picks up a bottle of the moscoto that Peggy likes. It'll help with the conversation. He makes a few other stops along the way to pick up some dinner and a movie. Mostly he just uses this time to window shop for the rest of the afternoon.

When he gets back to his apartment, Scott puts the wine and groceries into the refrigerator and begins making some spaghetti for dinner. Patty loves his spaghetti. His secret is the sauce and it's a simple one. He adds salsa to give it a little kick. He brings the pot of water to a boil and adds the oil and noodles and covers the pan. Scott then adds the sauce and salsa to a sauce pan and puts them on medium.

It's time. Scott is becoming more accepting of his medical condition. Going through it before was scary, but prepared him for this time. He had a lot of time to think about what dying would mean and knew that a recurrence was possible. Scott uses his cell phone to call his girls. It's not his plan to talk with them about this over the phone. That'll wait for this weekend when he sees them. But he wants to hear their voices.

"Hi baby, this is Dad." Scott greets Monica when she answers.

"Hi Daddy.." Monica and her father talk for about twenty minutes. Eventually she has to get off of the phone for dinner. Scott's is ready too and he bids her good night before briefly talking with his oldest Ellisa.

Scott hears the knock at the door and realizes the hour is later than he thought. Time flew by. He opens it to find Patty, standing at the door with a six pack of his favorite beer. He hugs her as she comes in and takes her coat.

Chapter 8

James brings Sara the envelope of labs from the state and reportable forms. Sara's opened up all of these every day since Scott turned this job over to her, but today is particularly difficult. As Sara flips through the stack of labs and report forms, one stands out among them. Katherine Johnson. Chris's little girl. The child's lab test comes back positive for gonorrhea. Sara's heart sinks as she holds the lab. There was no way for Sara or Scott to prevent the atrocity that the child had to endure. She separates the lab from the others and brings it down to Scott's office where she finds him watching a training video online. "Hi Sara, what's up?" Scott asks before he notices the melancholy expression. When he does, he turns off the web based training and motions for Sara to take a seat next to his desk.

"The lab reports came in." Sara says. The notification is unnecessary to her story, but she is compelled to begin with something simple. Sara can't think of a way to give Scott the news so she hands Scott the report instead of telling him.

Scott accepts the paper from Sara and sets it on the center of his desk. The room becomes quiet and the light seems to dim a little as he reads over the lab sheet. Sara is somewhat surprised to see that throughout, Scott remains stoic. Time slows, and it seems as though Scott takes an inordinate amount of time to comprehend. After he finishes reading he nods gently. "Now we know" is all he says. Scott then dials the Pediatric Clinic.

"Pediatric Clinic, how may I help you" the receptionists cheerful voice is antagonistic with the somber mood.

"May I speak with nurse Linda please, this is Scott at the health department."

"Yes, one moment please." Her tone is still overly cheery. The receptionist puts Scott on hold for a few minutes. The looped elevator music is occasionally interrupted by the recording of a woman's voice advising Scott that he is a valued customer and that they will be with him shortly.

"Hello, this is Linda." The nurse's voice is substantially less cheerful than that of the receptionist. Nurse Linda has been preparing to receive the laboratory report for the last couple of days, and she knows Scott never calls with good news.

"Hi Linda, this is Scott." Uncharacteristic for him he pauses before giving the nurse the news. This makes the receipt of it even harder. "We got Katharine's lab back today. It's positive for Gonorrhea.

"Oh God," Nurse Linda has taken care of Katharine since she was a baby. She's seen the child though some hard times. "Have you told the mother yet?"

Scott answers, but sounds very drained. "No, do you want me to call or do you want to? I can have her come to your clinic."

"Hmm, well I've already made a report to child welfare, maybe I'll have Dr. Hodge call them and see if the authorities can't pick up the child and bring her here for treatment." Nurse Linda seems much less skittish about calling the police on one of her patients now. Good. The girl will need some advocates.

"Sounds like a plan. Can you call me back and give me the treatment information?"

"I will, and thank you Scott."

The thanks is unnecessary, but appreciated. "Take care of yourself Linda. Good bye." Scott hangs up the phone and looks at Sara who has been glued to the conversation. "Thank you Sara." Scott's voice and being is muted. She isn't sure if the cause is his health, the stress from work, receiving the news about the child patient, or a combination of them. But she notices that he is not himself. Sara touches Scott's arm in a concerned gesture and walks out of his office.

"Can you close the door please?" He requests of Sara.

"Of course, call me if you need something." Sara closes the door behind her and walks towards her office.

Scott remembers the little girl's overwhelmed face and fearful posture from when she was in the clinic. The vision of her big brown eyes burns into his core. He remembers his interviewing Grimy, first at his nasty residence then again at the clinic. And he thinks about Chris and how miserable a mother would have to be to permit this nasty low life to harm her daughter. Scott sees people do the most horrible things to each other and at times it feels like all he does is help them do these things safer. Scott puts his hands over his face and sobs.

Sara walks down the now very familiar halls. A short time ago she didn't know how to navigate the clinic or even what she was doing here. Now, she feels like a part of this place. For better or worse, she is a part of the clinic. This investigation has been very hard. She's learned a lot about the practice of public health that couldn't be taught in a classroom. The world seems much larger and less abstract than it had. But she also feels tainted by touching the lives of people outside her experience. The prostitutes, the crack dealers, the convicts, and the child molesters have put a totally different face on this job than she ever knew existed. And now that she is aware, she's not sure this is for her. Does she want to become callous like Scott, spending decades in the filth trying to save the lives of people who don't appreciate her efforts? And look at what they do with this life. "No," Sara says to herself. "I'm not going to fight against the tide. I'm not going to end up like Scott." She enters her office and closes the door.

Epilogue

The Dr. calls child welfare and insists that they remove the child immediately from the home. The social service worker is accompanied by the police when she arrives at the apartment. She knocks on the door and Chris answers. "Hello?" Chris greets the officials while wearing an open robe with nothing underneath. Her hair is undone and she stammers while trying to ambulate. She appears to be high, intoxicated, or both. Behind her the officers can see the children watching TV. The house is filled with a rank smoke and stinks of old laundry. Upon seeing the officers Chris fumbles to close her robe, her cigarette still dangling from her lips.

"Chris Johnson?" Officer Larry says, "You're under arrest, please turn around and put your hands behind your head. Chris acts outraged and protests adamantly. Ironically, the children barely look away from the TV as their mother is placed into custody.

Chris is arrested for child abuse, felony drug possession, and prostitution. Her children are thankfully taken from her and placed into child welfare custody until suitable permanent placement can be found. Even though it's her first offense, the judge throws the book at her. She receives the maximum sentences allowed by law.

***

Red takes the advice of the social worker and enters drug treatment. He learns a lot about himself and finds his kids are the reason to improve his life.

They need to have a better chance than he had. Drug treatment gives Eddie a chance to get away from the lifestyle that consumed him since he was a child. Sobriety allows for Eddie's thoughts to clear. At first it's very hard. Drug and alcohol withdrawals were painfully difficult to get through. The sickness, confusion, and constant cravings makes it almost impossible to concentrate on anything else. As much as the loss of the addictive substances hurt, the loss of everything he knew and everyone he knew is also very hard to get past. Eddie realizes that if he is going to be successful he will have to reinvent himself. He will need completely different friends. The friends from his old life will only suck him back into that dark place where he knows he doesn't want to go again. Eddie also knows from talking with the drug treatment counselors, that he will need to find a different place to live. People know him in that building and even if he manages to stay away from his old friends, his acquaintances will come find him quickly.

Eddie credits divine intervention with his lack of a felony criminal record. During his life he's done so many illegal things it's amazing that he was never caught doing something serious. He's hurt a great number of people through his robbing, drug dealing, and numerous other crimes, some of which make him shudder to remember. Perhaps the real divine intervention is that he was never killed by a pissed off customer, competitor, police, or other disreputable person. Maybe God has a bigger plan for him.

Eddie does all that he's been asked to do during drug rehabilitation. He's well liked by the staff and makes some friends while he's in there. He even considers, albeit briefly, becoming a counselor himself. He completes the program and takes up the offer for job placement and housing assistance. He decides once he's back on his feet he'll try to get custody of his kids. He misses them and knows they need a loving parent to look after them.

After leaving rehab the workforce center helps him land a job as a janitor for the city working in a recreation center. The job is not high profile or particularly profitable, but the work is rewarding and Red is ideally situated to help young people stay away from the self destructive path that almost cost him everything. He gets along well with the customers, management, and coworkers. As he ages he's regarded as that old cat who's been there by some of the young kids in the neighborhood. And that's OK with Eddie.

Eddie's a good father and tries to teach his kids responsibility, treating people how they want to be treated, and the value of education and hard work. He makes a lot of mistakes as a parent, but his kids know that he loves them and will protect them. They trust him, and in this life, trust can be hard to come by. Red never uses crack again, but he smokes a little marijuana from time to time. Hey, it's risk reduction.

**

Over the next few months Scott becomes sicker. He begins to work half days, then eventually he is forced to resign. Peggy also takes a lot of time off from work so that she can care for Scott at his home while he goes though the chemotherapy treatment. Scott's daughters are broken hearted watching their father waste away. The oldest becomes very close to him as they mend their relationship.

On a bitterly cold morning, Ann enters the clinic. Her mood is heavy and somber. She passes the reception desk, past the office that still has Scott's name on the door, and upstairs to her own. Ann turns on her computer as she sits at her desk. Opening the e mail program she begins to compose a message to the staff.

"Yesterday, Scott Howard passed at his home. Even though he was very sick this comes as a shock to us all. Scott is survived by his two daughters, father, brother, and close friend Patty. Funeral services are to be announced. Please take this time to give your sympathies to them."

Ann knows that the message is short, but she's not sure what else to say. She'll take the next couple of days to think about it and provide words that do justice to her friend's life at a later time. For now, the employees at the clinic will grieve no matter how she tells them.

***

One morning at the clinic, Sara enters as she always does by greeting the staff and checking the mail. She's picked up a coffee habit from somewhere, but she's not sure how. She's always hated coffee. She removes the coffee cup with the clinic logo from her desk and brings it upstairs to the lounge. There, she sees nurse Marge eating some oatmeal with brown sugar and raisins. "Good morning Marge," Sara greets the nurse with a smile as she helps herself to the special brew. "How's it going?"

Marge looks up from her paper, happier than usual and reciprocates the greeting. "I'm great. It's a beautiful day for justice."

The response is perplexing to Sara who now looks inquisitively at Marge. "Come again?"

Marge sips her coffee with a thoroughly satisfied look on her face. "Check out page six of this morning's paper." The nurse slides the folded newspaper to the young woman with pleasure.

Sara picks up the newspaper from the lobby table. She usually doesn't bother to read the paper, preferring instead to get her news from network television. But the paper is folded over to display an article on the sixth page. The title catches Sara's attention "Thug Dies Like Thug." Her first thought is that the writer of the article and the editor really need lessons in sympathy. This completely lacks respect for someone who died. But, out of curiosity she lifts the paper to allow for proper reading of the article.

"At 2AM police responded to a call from the VIP lounge where a body was discovered. The body, belonging to Lawrence "Grimy" Polk, was found by residents and identified by family members later that morning. Police say Lawrence was found beaten to death with a brick that was found near the body.

Autopsy results indicated that the victim, Mr. Polk, did not die immediately from the injuries. Police stated that he attempted to make at least two phone calls for help, and crawled along the dirty alleyway for several meters, before succumbing to the fatal attack. The toxicology report indicated that the 'victim' had cocaine and alcohol in his system at the time of death.

Prior to the attack, Lawrence was patronizing the VIP lounge (a local strip club). The police report states that he was killed during a robbery, although no witnesses were found, and no suspects were arrested.

Lawrence "Grimy" Polk was wanted by police for his alleged involvement in narcotics sales, prostitution, and child sex abuse. He had previously evaded attempts by authorities to question him."

The nurses' earlier comments becoming extraordinarily clear, Sara sets the paper down. "Wow," She responds "that's amazing." She isn't sure what else to say about the news of this man's death. On one hand her civility demands that she not rejoice in the misfortunes of others, but on the other hand she believes that he got what he deserved. "Justice indeed."

Nurse Marge, still appearing very satisfied elects to use the Good Book to describe the events. She quoted Scripture stating "you live by the sword, you die by the sword." And nods her head acknowledging that it is God's will that this man was killed.

Sara's not as sure about it being divine will that struck down the late Mr. Polk. She can't deny that karma seems to be at play when bad things happen to bad people. But this may have been a case of the chickens coming home to roost. In any case, he won't function as a core transmitter in any other outbreaks, and that works out fine for Sara.

Sara takes her coffee and leaves the lounge for Ann's office. Ann's door is open and Sara knocks on the wall. The director looks up from her computer screen and motions Sara to come in. "Come in Sara, have a seat."

Sara complies and walks into the office. Sara notices that the office is darker than usual. Ann appears to have been here for a while based on the look of her desk. Papers are spread out, some in piles, others straggling between the piles as if they are lost children.

"Ann, I just want you to know that I've decided." Sara's decision was not an easy one. It really came down to how she sees herself and what impact she chooses to have on the world though her work.

Ann makes eye contact with Sara making sure that she's aware that the young employee has her full attention. "Sara, I know we've asked a lot of you, especially since you are so new here. And I know that the transition hasn't been easy for you. I want you to know that we really appreciate everything you've done. With Scott gone you've had to take on all of the responsibilities for the disease investigations at this health department. It's a hard, often times thankless job. But you've been great at it and if you need a reference please consider using me. It would be my pleasure to recommend you."

Sara has to fight back the tears. It has been hard. She's been here for a few months now and is basically alone. This isn't where she wanted to be.

She didn't go to school to work with STD's. Frankly, she didn't even know this job existed until she ran across the position post at the school. But none of that matters now. She is here. And the forces that brought her here did so for a reason. And now, with uncanny clarity she understands that reason.

"I'm staying." Sara announces to her boss. "Weird as it sounds, this is where I belong." The smile is as much from contentment with the situation as it is knowing that every day will bring its own rewards. As a disease investigator, Sara won't have to wait for a quarterly report or audit to know if she's made a difference. She won't need a power point presentation with graphs and charts. She'll know she's made a difference every day by the lives she touches. And that's why she chooses public health.

"I'm glad to hear it." The words don't do the sentiment justice. Ann knows that Sara is an irreplaceable member of the clinic and her staying means that the health department retains an incredibly valuable soldier in the fight against disease spread.

"I'm going to get back to it. We'll talk some more later." Sara stands from the chair and Ann replies, "I look forward to it."

Ann looks to the bookcase where a fresh picture rests. The image is of Scott and her husband, William, at a fishing trip in Tahoe a few years ago. They are both sitting in a rented fishing boat with the typical vests and boots. Scott is wearing too much sunscreen covering his face in a white pasty film. She smiles as she remembers the trip. Neither of them takes enough time off, but when they did, they had a times to remember. Sara deeply misses Scott. The hole that was left will never really be filled.

Sara goes back downstairs to her office and sits at her desk. The top is cluttered with stacks of piles of lab forms, case report forms, faxes, and investigation notes. But the pile that concerns her the most is just right of her keyboard. She takes the pile and moves it to the center of her desk and flips through the many forms, notes, and labs within. She documents the death of Lawrence Polk, also known as "Grimy." She adds the cases to the other folders and closes them.

Sara swivels her chair around to face three, four drawer file cabinets that were moved from Scott's office. She takes the stack of case folders and begins filing them appropriately. As she opens the drawers, Sara notices the many files identical to the ones she has just closed. So many lives touched by disease. She mourns the loss of her friend and teacher Scott. Sara closes the drawer and swivels around to face her desk again.

Sara surveys the stacks of piles around her desk, mentally inventorying them and prioritizing. She picks up a case report form that came in yesterday late afternoon. The gentleman tested positive for HIV from the hospital emergency room. Sara picks up the phone and calls the hospital.

"Emergency room, how may I help you?"

"Hi, this is Sara with the health department, may I speak with the charge nurse?"

***

Investigations end when everyone is either taken care of, refuses care, or can't be located. But, infections continue to spread. Sara will do all that she can until she's exhausted every lead, checked, and rechecked every case. Eventually this trail will go cold, but new trails will begin and the process will continue, forever. While at times it seems like she is fighting against the tide, Sara knows without a doubt that the work she does makes a difference. The people who don't get infected will never know to thank her, and she's OK with that. We don't do this to get rich or famous, Scott would say. We do it to protect our communities. And in the end, that's enough.

THE END

Thank you for reading this book. I've typed the words, but this story belongs to the women and men who work in the trenches to protect society from disease. Their dedication, knowledge, and professionalism make the world a safer place for all of us. And since they almost never hear it, I'd like to thank all of them for the work they have done. As for the work they are going to do...well, let's save some lives.

About the Author

I begin in public health as a Preventive Medicine Technician in the US Navy. The high quality education I received there has been an excellent foundation for everything I've learned and done since.

I attended Southern Illinois University at Carbondale (Salukies) and received a Bachelor of Science degree in Health Care Management (2002); and I have a Masters of Public Health degree from American Military University (2012).

I was a Disease Intervention Specialist for 8 years. As I am completing the final edits of this book my current position grants me the privilege of supervising an excellent disease investigative staff. As a manager I am able to enjoy many excellent stories and appreciate the impact that the staff has on disease through their investigations.

www.ingramcontent.com/pod-product-compliance
Lightning Source LLC
Chambersburg PA
CBHW051457170526
45166CB00001B/277